ALZHEIMER'S DIET COOKBOOK FOR SENIORS

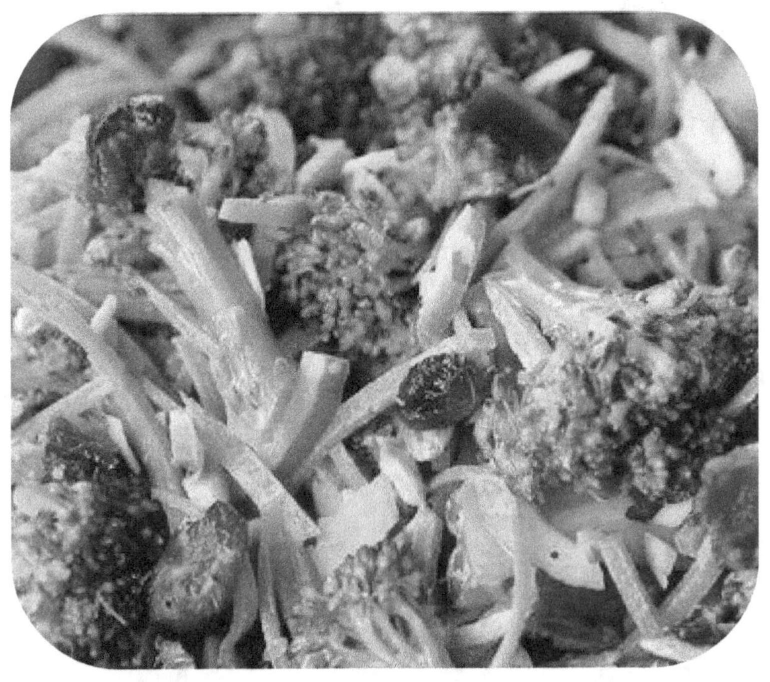

2000 DAYS OF QUICK, EASY AND DELICIOUS BRAIN BOOSTING RECIPES TO HELP PREVENT MEMORY DISORDERS, ALZHEIMER'S & DEMENTIA FOR A HEALTHY LIFE (WITH 98 DAYS MEAL PLAN)

CARLY EVELYN

SCAN TO GET MORE BOOKS BY THIS AUTHOR

IF YOU ARE STUCK, WHILE PREPARING ANY RECIPES IN THIS COOKBOOK, YOU CAN REACH THE AUTHOR AT CARLYEVLCUISINEGUIDE@GMAIL.COM FOR GUIDANCE

TABLE OF CONTENT

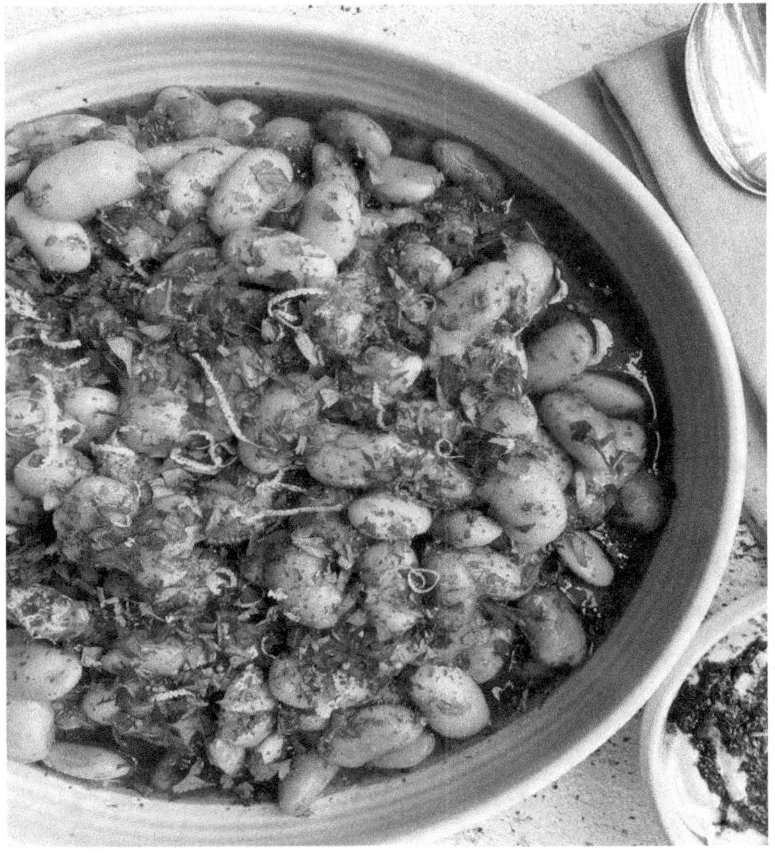

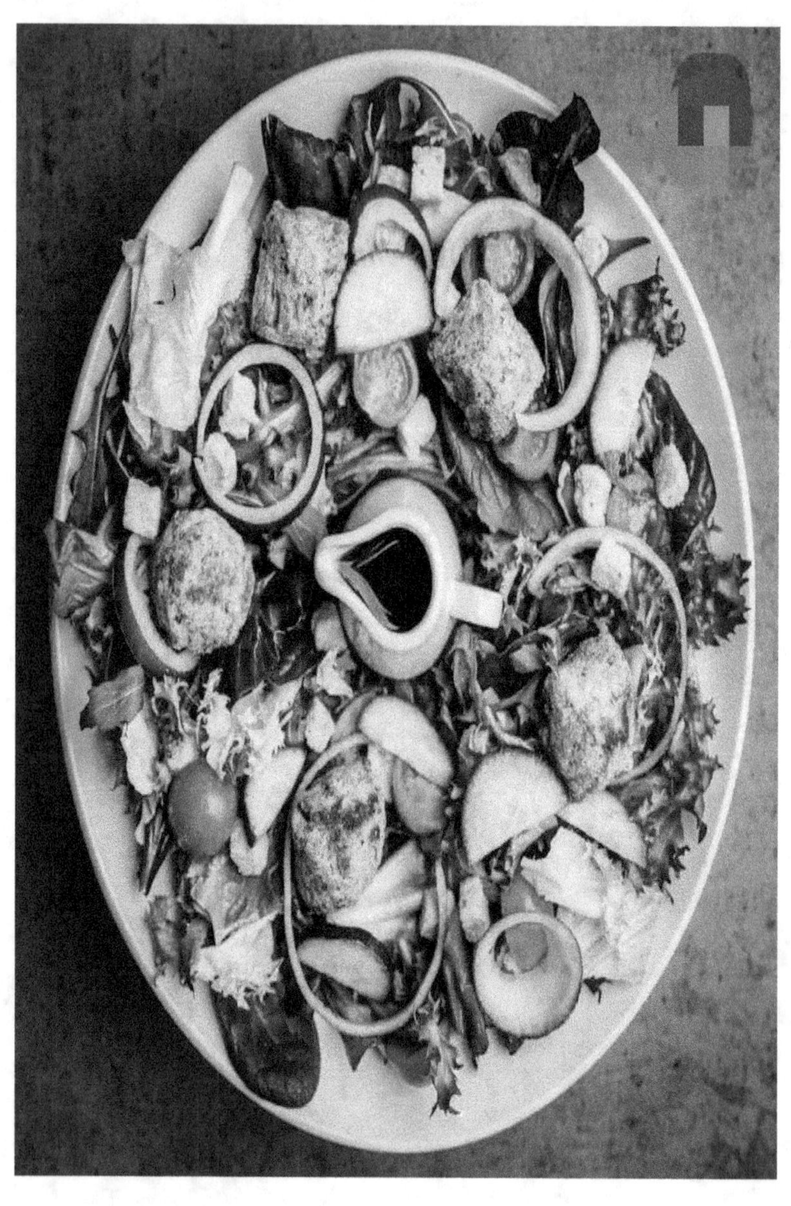

INTRODUCTION

In the heart of the charming city of Asheville, nestled amid the breathtaking Blue Ridge Mountains, lived a close-knit community of seniors in a peaceful retirement home. Among them was Margaret, a vibrant and spirited woman who had once been a renowned nutritionist. As the years went by, Margaret noticed a subtle decline in her cognitive abilities, a cloud that seemed to dim the brilliance of her mind. Eventually, she received a devastating diagnosis: early-stage Alzheimer's disease.

Refusing to surrender to the inevitable, Margaret delved into research and rediscovered her passion for nutrition. She became determined to explore the profound impact of diet on brain health. With unwavering resolve, she crafted a comprehensive plan that focused on foods known for their cognitive benefits.

Margaret's plan included a variety of nutrient-dense foods such as leafy greens, berries rich in antioxidants, fatty fish abundant in omega-3 fatty acids, and nuts packed with brain-boosting nutrients. She incorporated these elements into delicious and meticulously planned meals, advocating for a diet that nourished not only the body but also the mind.

As word spread about Margaret's journey and her newfound dedication to nutrition, her fellow seniors joined her in this culinary adventure. The retirement home's dining hall transformed into a hub of excitement and camaraderie as residents shared recipes, swapped cooking tips, and eagerly embraced their new dietary regimen.

The community thrived on the sense of purpose and connection that Margaret's initiative brought. Friends who had once experienced the fog of forgetfulness found themselves engaged in vibrant conversations and rediscovered the joy of shared memories. The once-dreaded specter of Alzheimer's seemed to loosen its grip, and hope blossomed among the residents.

Months passed, and the transformation was remarkable. Margaret, once a victim of the insidious effects of Alzheimer's, now exuded vitality. She navigated the streets of Asheville with a newfound clarity, appreciating the beauty of the mountains as if seeing them for the first time. Her fellow seniors, too, marveled at the improvements in their cognitive abilities and relished the sense of accomplishment that came with overcoming the challenges of aging.

News of this extraordinary feat reached not only the local community but also the broader medical community. Margaret became an unwitting beacon of inspiration for those seeking alternative approaches to managing Alzheimer's disease.

In the heart of Asheville, against the backdrop of the serene Blue Ridge Mountains, a community of seniors defied the odds, proving that with the right diet and a collective spirit, they could reverse or manage the grasp of Alzheimer's disease. Margaret's journey became a testament to the power of resilience, community, and the transformative potential of the food we choose to nourish our bodies and minds.

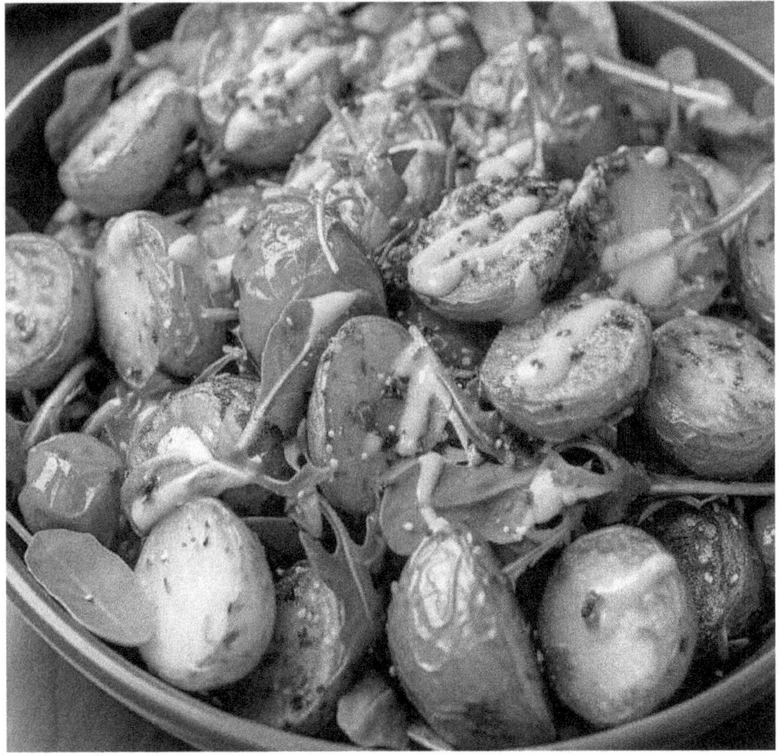

FOODS TO EAT OR AVOID ON AN ALZHEIMER'S DISEASE DIET TO ACHIEVE OPTIMUM HEALTH.

A well-balanced diet is essential for maintaining overall health, and this is particularly true for those suffering from Alzheimer's disease. While there is no treatment for Alzheimer's, a well-balanced diet may improve general health and perhaps decrease cognitive deterioration. The Alzheimer's disease diet emphasizes nutrient-dense foods that promote brain function, contain antioxidants, and decrease inflammation. In this section, we'll look at which foods to eat and which to avoid if you want to stay healthy while dealing with Alzheimer's.

RECOMMENDED FOODS:

1. Fatty Fish: Omega-3 fatty acids, which may be found in salmon, trout, and sardines, are essential for brain function. These fatty acids are anti-inflammatory and help with cognitive function.

2. Bright Fruits and Vegetables: Antioxidants are abundant in berries, leafy greens, and vividly colored vegetables. These molecules aid in the fight against oxidative stress, which has been related to cognitive deterioration.

3. Nuts and Seeds: Omega-3 fatty acids, antioxidants, and protein are abundant in walnuts, almonds, flaxseeds, and chia seeds. They boost general brain function and give long-lasting energy.

4. Whole Grains: Foods like brown rice, whole wheat bread, and quinoa provide the brain with a consistent flow of energy. They also provide fiber, which promotes gastrointestinal health, which is connected to cognitive function.

5. Lean Proteins: Chicken, turkey, lean beef, and plant-based proteins such as lentils and tofu provide essential amino acids for brain function. Proteins are also involved in the synthesis of neurotransmitters.

Healthy Fats: Healthy monounsaturated fats found in olive oil, avocado, and coconut oil promote cardiovascular health. Maintaining brain health requires a healthy heart.

Turmeric: Turmeric's main ingredient, curcumin, has anti-inflammatory and antioxidant properties. Turmeric may help battle the inflammation linked with Alzheimer's disease.

8. Low-Fat Dairy: Low-fat dairy products such as yogurt and milk include critical minerals such as calcium and vitamin D, which are needed for bone health and general well-being.

Herbs and spices: Other herbs, such as rosemary and sage, have been linked to possible cognitive advantages. They give flavor to recipes without adding too much salt.

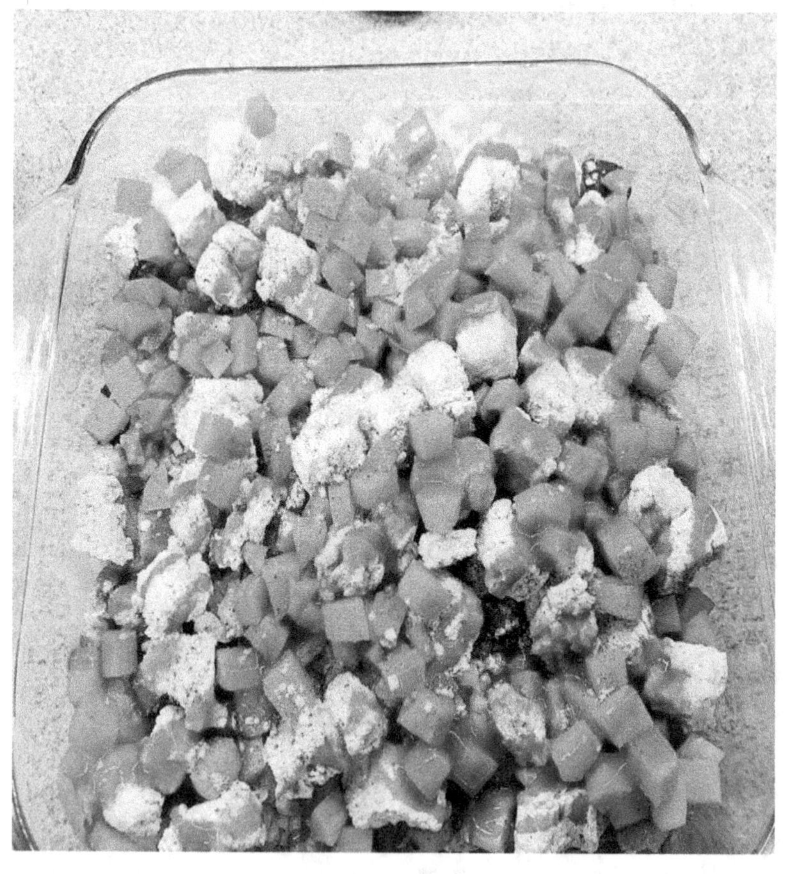

1. Manufactured Foods: Trans fats, high salt levels, and artificial additives are common in highly processed diets. These may cause inflammation and have a detrimental impact on general health.

Saturated and Trans Fats: It is critical to limit your consumption of saturated fats found in butter, full-fat dairy, and processed meats. Trans fats, which are often found in fried and baked items, may lead to inflammation and heart disease.

3. Sugars Added: Diets rich in added sugars are linked to increased inflammation and an increased risk of acquiring chronic diseases. Sugary meals and drinks should be avoided at all costs.

4. Excessive alcohol consumption: While moderate alcohol use may have certain health advantages, excessive alcohol consumption has been linked to cognitive deterioration. It is critical to stick to the suggested limits.

Highly Salted Foods: Excessive salt consumption may cause high blood pressure, which has a detrimental influence on vascular health. Hidden salt is often found in processed meals and snacks.

6. Full-Fat Dairy: Consuming a lot of full-fat dairy products might raise your cholesterol levels. Choose low-fat or fat-free options.

7. Carbohydrates that have been refined: White bread, spaghetti, and other refined carbs may cause blood sugar spikes, which can impair cognitive performance over time. Choose whole grains for long-lasting energy.

Finally, Alzheimer's disease diet focuses on nutrient-dense, complete foods that promote brain function and general well-being. Focus on a range of colorful fruits and vegetables, lean proteins, healthy fats, and whole grains, while avoiding processed meals, added sweets, and excessive salt.

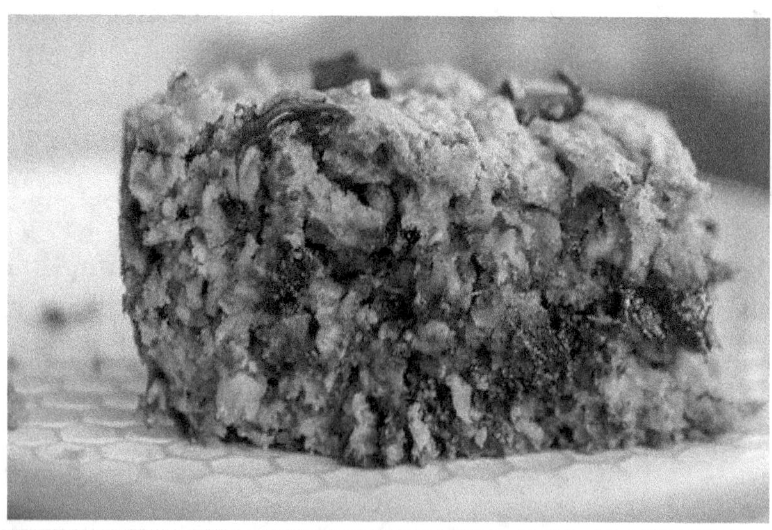

CORE BENEFITS OF FOLLOWING AN ALZHEIMER'S DISEASE DIET FOR SENIORS.

Following an Alzheimer's disease diet may provide numerous key advantages for seniors, especially those suffering from cognitive impairment. This specialized diet emphasizes nutrient-dense foods that promote brain health, offer critical vitamins and minerals, and aid in the management of Alzheimer's disease symptoms. Here are some of the primary advantages of following an Alzheimer's disease diet for seniors:

1. Cognitive Support: - Nutritional Foods: Foods high in omega-3 fatty acids, antioxidants, and critical elements that enhance cognitive function are included in the diet. Omega-3 fatty acids present in fish contribute to brain function, and antioxidants assist counteract oxidative stress, which has been related to cognitive decline.

2. Reduced Inflammation: - Anti-Inflammatory Foods: The diet is intended to minimize inflammation, which has been linked to the development of Alzheimer's disease. Anti-inflammatory foods include fatty fish, nuts, seeds, and colored fruits and vegetables.

3. Cardiovascular Health: - Healthy Fats: Healthy fats, such as those found in olive oil, avocados, and almonds, are beneficial to cardiovascular health. Maintaining appropriate blood flow to the brain requires a healthy heart.

4. Regulation of Blood Sugar: - Whole Grains and Low-Glycemic Foods: The diet emphasizes whole grains and restricts processed carbs, which aids with blood sugar regulation. Blood sugar levels that are stable contribute to general well-being and may minimize the risk of cognitive impairment.

5. Balanced Nutrition: - Weight Management: The diet encourages a well-rounded, balanced dietary intake, which may help with weight control. Maintaining a healthy weight is essential for general health and lowering the risk of chronic diseases.

6. Better Gut Health: - Fiber-Rich Foods: Fiber from fruits, vegetables, and whole grains is beneficial to intestinal health. New study indicates a link between intestinal health and brain performance.

7. Bone Health: Calcium and Vitamin D: Low-fat dairy products provide calcium and vitamin D, which are needed for bone health. This is especially crucial for elderly who may be prone to osteoporosis.

8. Reduced Chronic Disease Risk: - Whole Foods: The diet leads to a lower risk of chronic illnesses such as diabetes and cardiovascular difficulties by concentrating on natural, minimally processed foods and minimizing added sugars and bad fats.

9. Attention to Hydration: - Water-Rich Foods: Many items in the Alzheimer's disease diet, such as fruits and vegetables, include a lot of water, which helps with hydration. Hydration is critical for general health and well-being.

10. Potential Symptom Management: - Nutritional Influence on Symptoms: While not a cure, an Alzheimer's disease diet may help control some of the condition's symptoms. Including meals high in particular nutrients, for example, may improve mood and reduce certain behavioral problems.

11. Improved Quality of Life: - Overall Well-Being: The combination of cognitive support, lower inflammation, and higher nutritional intake results in an improved quality of life for seniors who follow an Alzheimer's disease diet.

Individual reactions to dietary treatments may vary, and the Alzheimer's disease diet is not a one-size-fits-all solution. It is critical to consult with healthcare specialists, particularly registered dietitians, in order to adapt dietary advice based on individual health condition, preferences, and requirements.

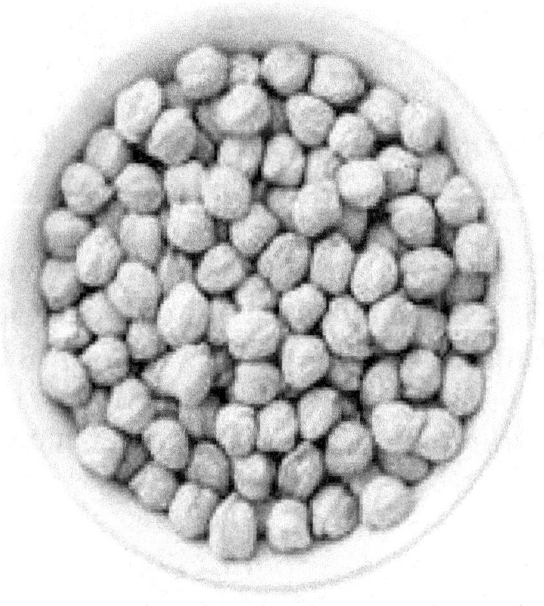

Chickpeas

20 HEALTHY SHOPPING INGREDIENTS OR LISTS FOR AN ALZHEIMER'S DISEASE DIET.

Making a grocery list for an Alzheimer's diet entails choosing nutrient-dense foods that promote brain health and general well-being. Here are 20 healthful Alzheimer's diet buying ingredients:

1. Fatty Fish: Salmon, Trout, Sardines: Omega-3 fatty acids, which promote brain function.

2. Bright Fruits: Blueberries, Strawberries, Oranges: Antioxidant-rich to counteract oxidative stress.

3. Leafy Greens: Spinach, Kale, and Swiss Chard Folate, vitamins, and antioxidants are abundant.

4. Nuts: Walnuts and Almonds: Give omega-3 fatty acids, antioxidants, and healthy fats.

5. Seeds: Flaxseeds, Chia Seeds: Omega-3s, fiber, and antioxidants are abundant.

6. Whole Grains: Quinoa, Brown Rice, Oats: Maintain energy and necessary nutrients.

7. Lean Proteins: Chicken, Turkey, Tofu: It is required for the creation of amino acids and neurotransmitters.

8. Healthy Fats: Olive Oil, Avocado, and Coconut Oil: Monounsaturated fats are beneficial to cardiovascular health.

9. Turmeric: (Ground or Fresh) Curcumin, which has anti-inflammatory and antioxidant effects, is present.

10. Low-Fat Dairy: Greek Yogurt, Skim Milk: Calcium and vitamin D source for bone health.

11. Herbs and spices: Rosemary, Sage, Cinnamon: Add flavor without using too much salt or sugar.

12. Broccoli: High in Antioxidants: It promotes general wellness and contains fiber.

13. Cauliflower: Adaptable: Can be used to make a variety of foods, including cauliflower rice.

14. Berries: Strawberries and Raspberries: Antioxidants and vitamins abound.

15. Beans and Legumes: Chickpeas and Lentils: Protein, fiber, and necessary nutrients should be included.

16. Tomatoes: Lycopene-rich: A strong antioxidant with possible cognitive effects.

17. Bell Peppers: Vibrant and Nutrient-Dense: Vitamin and antioxidant content is high.

18. Sweet Potatoes: Source of Beta-Carotene: It promotes general health and gives you energy.

19. Eggs: High in Choline: Brain health and neurotransmitter function are both dependent on it.

20. Low-Sodium Broth: Vegetable or Chicken: Excellent for making nutrient-dense soups.

When shopping for an Alzheimer's diet, prefer whole foods over processed meals and fresh, seasonal vegetables wherever feasible. It's also a good idea to eat a variety of meals to get a wide range of nutrients

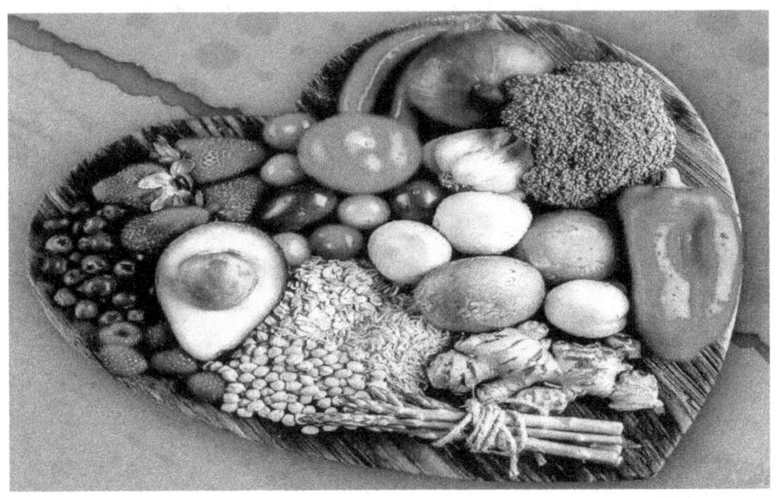

COMPLICATIONS OF ALZHEIMER'S DISEASE, IF THE RIGHT DIET ISN'T ADOPTED.

While eating a nutritious diet may help people with Alzheimer's disease feel better, it's vital to remember that food alone cannot prevent or cure the illness. However, failing to follow a healthy diet may lead to a variety of issues and increase Alzheimer's symptoms. Here are several difficulties that may emerge if patients with Alzheimer's do not follow the proper diet:

1. **Malnutrition:** Alzheimer's patients may struggle with meal preparation, remembering to eat, or experiencing changes in appetite. This may result in insufficient nutrition and malnutrition, which can contribute to weakness, weight loss, and general health deterioration.

2. **Cognitive Decline:** Poor diet, especially a lack of vital nutrients, might possibly hasten cognitive decline in people with Alzheimer's disease. The brain needs sufficient nourishment to operate properly, and dietary deficits may have a severe influence on cognitive functions.

Increased Behavioral Symptoms: Inadequate nutrition may contribute to the increased behavioral and psychological symptoms of Alzheimer's disease, such as agitation, anger, and mood swings. These symptoms may exacerbate caring and reduce an individual's quality of life.

4. Impaired Immune Function: Malnutrition may impair the immune system, rendering people more vulnerable to infections and other health problems. Infections, such as urinary tract infections, are frequent in Alzheimer's patients and may exacerbate cognitive and behavioral symptoms.

5. Bone Health Issues: Deficiencies in minerals such as calcium and vitamin D may lead to bone health problems such as osteoporosis and an increased risk of fractures. This is especially important for Alzheimer's patients who are already at risk for bone abnormalities.

6. Dehydration: Individuals with Alzheimer's disease may overlook their hydration requirements due to forgetfulness or communication issues. Dehydration may cause major health concerns such as urinary tract infections, renal difficulties, and a higher chance of falling.

7. Medication Interactions: Some drugs regularly administered for Alzheimer's patients may have dietary limitations or interactions. Failure to follow these rules may reduce the medication's efficacy or cause undesired side effects.

Gastrointestinal Problems: Constipation and other gastrointestinal issues may be exacerbated by poor diet. Furthermore, a lack of dietary fiber may worsen digestive difficulties typical in Alzheimer's patients.

9. Cardiovascular Complications: Poor eating habits might lead to cardiovascular problems such as high blood pressure and high cholesterol levels. Cardiovascular health is inextricably connected to general health and cognitive function.

10. Increased Caregiver Stress: The difficulties involved with managing someone with Alzheimer's nutritional requirements, particularly if they avoid eating or have trouble conveying their preferences, may dramatically raise caregiver stress.

Individuals with Alzheimer's disease and their caregivers must collaborate closely with healthcare specialists, particularly registered dietitians, to establish and execute a personalized dietary plan. Regular medical check-ups, monitoring nutritional status, and making required dietary modifications are all important components of complete Alzheimer's treatment. Addressing the varied requirements of people with Alzheimer's requires a multidisciplinary approach that involves healthcare practitioners, caregivers, and nutrition specialists.

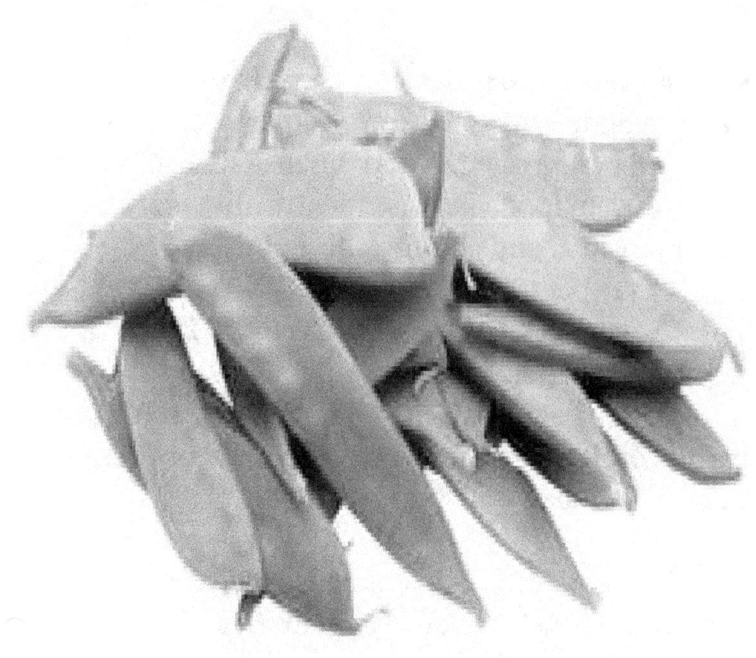

Snow Peas

MEAL PLANNING FOR ALZHEIMER'S DISEASE DIET, HIGHLIGHTING ITS BENEFITS FOR PROPER MANAGEMENT.

Meal planning for an Alzheimer's disease diet entails carefully selecting nutrient-dense meals that promote brain health and general well-being. This planning is especially crucial since people with Alzheimer's may have memory problems, hunger changes, and food preparation issues. Here's a guide to Alzheimer's meal planning, as well as its advantages for effective management:

Alzheimer's Meal Planning:

1. A well-balanced nutrient intake: Plan meals that are high in macronutrients (carbohydrates, proteins, and fats) and low in micronutrients (vitamins and minerals). This ensures that the body and brain get the nutrients they need for optimum operation.

2. Regular and Consistent Meals: Create a regimen that includes regular meal times. Meal plan consistency helps people with Alzheimer's anticipate and remember when it's time to eat, minimizing confusion and anxiety.

3. Range of Foods: Include a range of colorful fruits and vegetables, lean meats, complete grains, and healthy fats in your diet. A varied diet contains a variety of nutrients and antioxidants that are advantageous to brain function.

4. Hydration: Ensure that you drink enough fluids throughout the day. Dehydration may increase cognitive issues, so keep water and other hydrating liquids nearby.

5. Finger-Friendly meals: Think about include finger-friendly or easy-to-eat meals. This is particularly useful if the client has trouble handling utensils or has motor skill issues.

6. Healthy Snacks: Plan healthy snacks in between meals. Snacks may help keep energy levels up while also providing extra opportunity to consume critical nutrients.

7. Culinary Familiarity: Include meals that the person is acquainted with. Taste and appearance familiarity may boost hunger and make eating more pleasurable.

8. Reduce Processed Foods: Reduce your intake of processed foods, refined carbohydrates, and harmful fats. To improve general health and well-being, prioritize whole, minimally processed meals.

9. Think About Texture Modifications: Depending on individual requirements, think about adjusting food textures. It may be necessary to change the consistency of meals to make them simpler to chew and swallow.

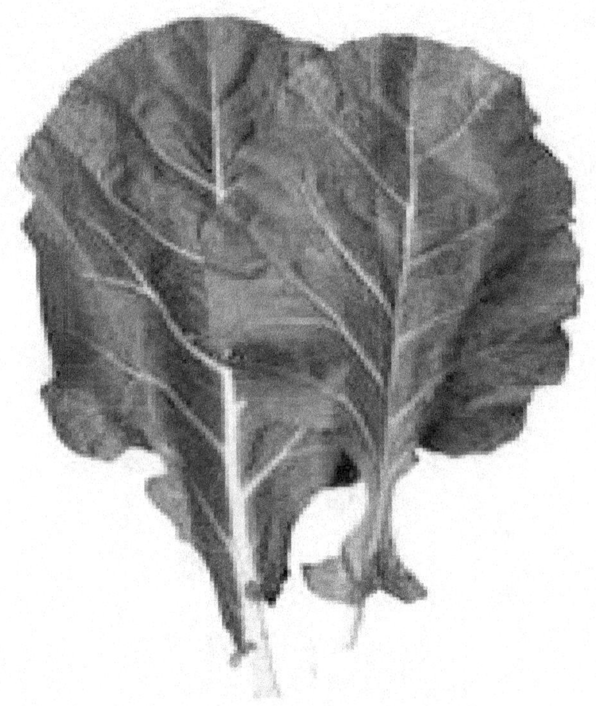

Collard Greens

Spaghetti Squash

BENEFITS OF MEAL PLANNING FOR ALZHEIMER'S DISEASE:

1. Nutritional Support: A well-planned diet ensures that people with Alzheimer's get the nutrients they need for good health and cognitive function. This dietary supplementation has the ability to delay cognitive deterioration.

2. Weight Management: Meal planning aids in the maintenance of a healthy weight. Adequate diet promotes general well-being and aids in the prevention of undesired weight loss or increase.

3. Improved Cognitive Function: Proper nutrition may improve cognitive function. Certain nutrients, such as omega-3 fatty acids and antioxidants, may help to maintain brain function and maybe slow cognitive loss.

4. Better Hydration: Incorporating hydrated meals and drinks into the meal plan helps avoid dehydration, which may impair cognitive and physical performance.

5. Predictability and schedule: Establishing a consistent mealtime schedule may help people with Alzheimer's disease avoid confusion and anxiety. Routine contributes to a feeling of order and normality.

6. Reduced Behavioral Symptoms: Adequate diet may help to reduce the behavioral symptoms linked with Alzheimer's disease. Reduced agitation or mood fluctuations may result from improved overall well-being.

7. Simplified Eating Experience: Choosing finger-friendly or easy-to-eat foods streamlines the eating experience, making it more pleasurable and less difficult for those with Alzheimer's disease.

8. Caregiver Support: Meal planning is an organized method that assists caregivers in addressing the dietary requirements of Alzheimer's patients. It may help to alleviate the stress associated with meal preparation and decision-making.

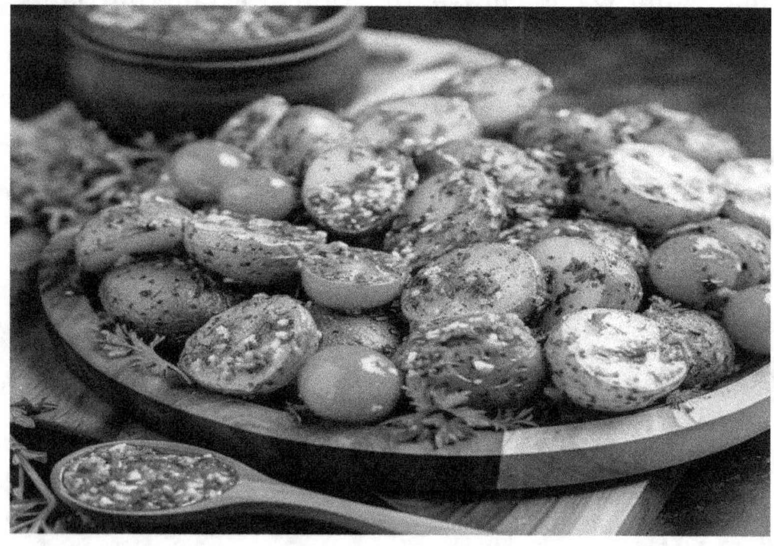

SERIAL 14-DAY SAMPLE ALZHEIMER'S DISEASE MEAL PLAN.

Developing a 28-day example meal plan for Alzheimer's disease entails including nutrient-dense meals, emphasizing variety, and taking into account elements like ease of preparation and cognitive support. This plan is just a recommendation and should be modified depending on personal tastes, dietary requirements, and any special concerns

Day 1

Breakfast:
- Greek yogurt parfait with mixed berries and walnut streusel
- Avocado on whole grain bread

Lunch:
- Salad with spinach and salmon with a variety of bright veggies
- Roasted veggie quinoa pilaf

Dinner:
- Lemon-herb baked chicken breast - Steamed broccoli and cauliflower - Quinoa and veggie stir-fry

Snack:
- Apple slices with almond butter

Day 2

Breakfast:
- Scrambled eggs with spinach and cherry tomatoes - Oatmeal with sliced bananas and honey drizzle

Lunch:
- Lentil and vegetable soup - Whole grain roll with mixed green salad on the side

Dinner:
- Grilled fish with dill and lemon sauce - Steamed asparagus - sweet potato and black bean bowl

Snack: Greek yogurt with fresh blueberries

Day 3

Breakfast:
- Strawberry and kiwi chia seed pudding - Whole grain pancakes with maple syrup

Lunch:
- Whole wheat tortilla wrap with turkey and avocado - Salad of mixed greens with a mild vinaigrette

Dinner:
- Tofu and veggies stir-fried with brown rice - Roasted Brussels sprouts with a balsamic glaze

Snack:
Trail mix with almonds and dried fruit

Day 4

Breakfast:
- Whole grain toast with sliced peaches and cottage cheese
- Omelette with spinach and mushrooms

Lunch:
- Stir-fry quinoa and veggies
- Granola and Greek yogurt parfait

Dinner:
- Baked rosemary and garlic chicken
- Stir-fry cauliflower "rice" with assorted veggies

Snack: Cottage cheese with slices of pineapple

Day 5

Breakfast:
- Quinoa with apple cinnamon - Scrambled eggs with chopped bell peppers

Lunch:
- Mediterranean chickpea salad - Whole grain hummus wrap

Dinner:
- Avocado-topped grilled turkey burgers
- Steamed green beans - Roasted sweet potatoes

Snack:
- Blueberry-almond crepe

Day 6

Breakfast:
- Smoothie of blueberries and bananas with Greek yogurt, almond milk, and chia seeds
- Strawberry whole grain waffle

Lunch:
- Vegetable and lentil stew
- Quinoa salad with cucumber and cherry tomatoes

Dinner:
- Quinoa-topped baked salmon - Stir-fried broccoli and snap peas - Mashed sweet potatoes

Snack:
- Greek yogurt with honey drizzle

Breakfast:
- Chia seeded banana ice cream
- Avocado with poached egg on whole grain bread

Lunch:
- Kebabs of turkey and vegetables with whole grain couscous
- Stuffed mushrooms with spinach and feta

Dinner:
- Quiche with spinach and mushrooms served with a side salad - Baked sweet potato wedges

Snack: Nut and dark chocolate trail mix

Day 8

Breakfast:
- Oatmeal with mixed berries and a dollop of Greek yogurt overnight
- Peach sliced whole grain pancakes

Lunch:
- Whole wheat tortilla wrap with chicken and vegetables
- Quinoa salad with cucumber and cherry tomatoes

Dinner:
- Garlic and lemon grilled shrimp
- Stir-fry with quinoa and vegetables
- Sautéed broccoli

Snack: Cottage cheese with slices of pineapple

Day 9

Breakfast:
- Smoothie with blueberries and kale, almond milk, and a scoop of protein powder
- Scrambled spinach and mushrooms

Lunch:
- Soup with lentils and vegetables - Whole grain roll with hummus

Dinner:
- Chicken baked with rosemary and lemon
- Sweet potato and black bean dish - Balsamic-glazed Brussels sprouts

Snack: Greek yogurt with a few almonds

Day 10

Breakfast:
- Mango and kiwi chia seed pudding - Strawberries on whole grain waffle

Lunch:
- Whole wheat tortilla wrap with turkey and avocado
- Roasted veggie quinoa pilaf

Dinner:
- Honey-mustard glazed grilled salmon
- Stir-fry cauliflower "rice" with assorted veggies

Snack:
- Apple slices with almond butter

Day 11

Breakfast:
- Greek yogurt parfait topped with mixed berries and oats - Scrambled eggs with sliced bell peppers

Lunch:
- Mediterranean chickpea salad - Whole grain hummus wrap

Dinner:

- Tofu and veggies stir-fried with brown rice - Roasted sweet potatoes - Steamed green beans

Snack:
Trail mix with almonds and dried fruit

Day 12

Breakfast:
- Quinoa dish with apple cinnamon - Whole grain toast with cottage cheese and sliced peaches

Lunch:
- Salad with spinach and salmon with a variety of bright veggies
- Quinoa salad with cucumber and cherry tomatoes

Dinner:
- Baked garlic and herb chicken - Quinoa and veggie stir-fry
- Broccoli and cauliflower steamed

Snack:
- Blueberry-almond crepe

Day 13

Breakfast:
- Chia seeded banana ice cream
- Avocado with poached egg on whole grain bread

Lunch:
- Vegetable and lentil stew
- Roasted veggie quinoa pilaf

Dinner:
- Avocado-topped grilled turkey burgers
- Balsamic-glazed roasted Brussels sprouts - Mashed sweet potatoes

Snack:
- Greek yogurt with honey drizzle

Day 14

Breakfast:
- Smoothie of blueberries and bananas with Greek yogurt and almond milk
- Omelette with spinach and mushrooms

Lunch:
- Whole wheat tortilla wrap with chicken and vegetables
- Salad of mixed greens with a mild vinaigrette

Dinner:
- Baked salmon over quinoa - Stir-fried broccoli and snap peas - Mango slices for dessert

Snack: Nut and dark chocolate trail mix

Continue in this manner, consuming a variety of meals and changing portion sizes as needed. It is critical to evaluate the individual's reaction to the meal plan, make any changes, and engage with healthcare specialists for continuous support and direction. Regular hydration and nutritious snacks between meals may also be included to provide the best nutritional assistance for you.

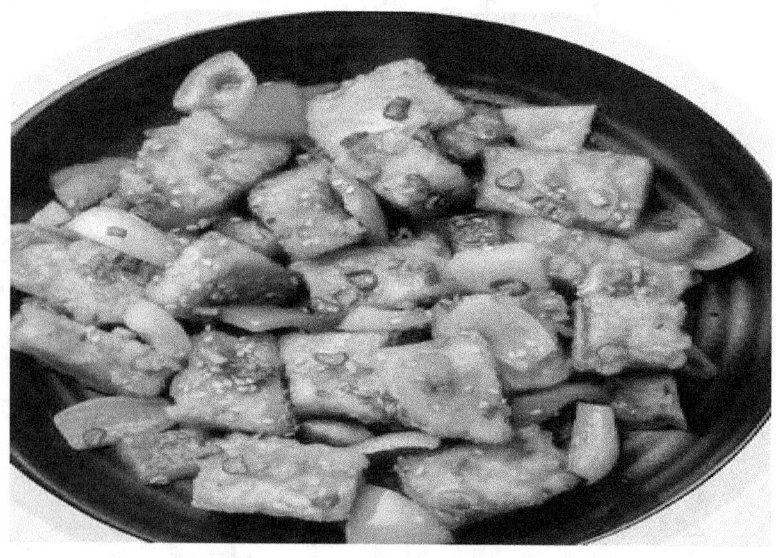

ALZHEIMER'S DISEASE BREAKFAST RECIPES

1. Berry Creamy Oatmeal

Ingredients:
- 1 cup rolled oats, old-fashioned - 2 cups water
- 1 cup berries (blueberries, strawberries, and raspberries)
2 tbsp honey 1/4 cup chopped nuts (almonds, walnuts)
- 1/2 teaspoon ground cinnamon
- 1/2 cup skim milk

Instructions:
1. Bring water to a boil in a saucepan.
2. Stir in the rolled oats and reduce to a low heat. Cook, stirring periodically, for 5-7 minutes, or until the oats are creamy.
3. Turn off the heat and stir in the mixed berries, honey, chopped almonds, cinnamon, and milk.
4. Give it a good stir and let aside for a minute to enable the berries to soften.
5. Serve warm and enjoy the nutritious delight.

Nutritional Factors:
- 400 calories
- 15g protein
- 8g fiber

- 10g of good fats
- Antioxidants: abundant

Preparation Time: 10 minutes

2.Greek Yogurt Parfait

Ingredients:
- 1 cup plain Greek yogurt
- 1 granola cup
1/2 cup mixed berries (strawberries, blueberries)
- 1/4 cup chopped almonds - 1 tablespoon honey

Instructions:
1. Layer Greek yogurt, granola, and mixed berries in a glass or dish.
2. Drizzle with honey and sprinkle with sliced almonds.
3. Continue with the layers.
4. Serve immediately to keep the granola crunchy.

Nutritional Factors:
- 350 calories
- 20g protein
- 6g fiber
- 15g of good fats
- Probiotics: abundant

Preparation Time: 5 Minutes

3. Scrambled Spinach and Mushrooms

Ingredients:
- 2 eggs
- 1 cup chopped fresh spinach
- 1/2 cup sliced mushrooms
1 teaspoon olive oil
- Season with salt and pepper to taste

Instructions:
1. In a pan over medium heat, heat the olive oil.
2. Sauté the mushrooms until tender.
3. Add the spinach and simmer until it has wilted.
4. In a mixing dish, whisk together the eggs and season with salt and pepper.
5. Pour the eggs over the veggies and gently stir until the eggs are fully cooked.
6. Serve immediately.

Nutritional Factors:
- 250 calories
- 15g protein
- 3g fiber
- 18g of healthy fat
- Vitamin K: abundant

Preparation Time: 10 minutes

4. Chia Seed Pudding:

Ingredients:
- 1 tablespoon chia seeds
1 cup of almond milk
-1 teaspoon honey
- 1/2 teaspoon vanilla essence
- Fresh fruit (kiwi, berries) for garnish

Instructions:
1. Combine chia seeds, almond milk, honey, and vanilla essence in a mixing dish.
2. Stir thoroughly and place in the fridge for at least 2 hours or overnight.
3. Before serving, re-stir the mixture and garnish with fresh fruit.

Nutritional Factors:
- 200 calories
- 5g protein
- 10g fiber
- 10g of good fats
- Omega-3 Fatty Acids: abundant

Time to Prepare: 5 minutes (plus chilling time)

5. Whole-Wheat Pancakes:

Ingredients:
1 cup whole wheat flour 1 tbsp baking powder
1 cup almond milk - 1 tbsp honey
- 1 egg
- 1/2 tsp vanilla extract
- Fresh fruit (bananas, blueberries) for garnish

Instructions:
1. Whisk together whole wheat flour, baking powder, honey, almond milk, egg, and vanilla extract in a mixing dish until smooth.
2. Melt butter on a griddle or nonstick pan over medium heat.
3. Pour 1/4 cup batter onto the griddle for each pancake.
4. Cook until surface bubbles appear, then turn and cook the other side.
5. Garnish with fresh fruit.

Nutritional Factors:
- 300 calories
- 10g protein
- 6g fiber
- 5g of healthy fat

Preparation Time: 15 Minutes

6. Veggie Breakfast Burrito

Ingredients:
- 1 whole-wheat tortilla
- 2 scrambled eggs
- 1/4 cup washed and drained black beans
- 1 tablespoon chopped tomatoes
- 1/4 cup bell peppers, diced
- 1 tablespoon shredded cheese
- Salsa for sprinkling

Instructions:
1. Preheat the tortilla on a dry skillet or in the microwave.
2. Scramble the eggs in a separate pan until they are done.
3. Layer the scrambled eggs, black beans, tomatoes, bell peppers, and shredded cheese on top of the tortilla. Roll the tortilla up and top with salsa.

Nutritional Factors:
- 400 calories
- 20g protein
- 8g fiber
- 15g of good fats
- Vitamin C: abundant

Preparation Time: 10 minutes

7. Apple Cinnamon Quinoa Bowl

Ingredients:
- 1 cup water
- 1/2 cup quinoa
- 1 diced apple
- 1/2 teaspoon ground cinnamon
- 2 tbsp. pecans, chopped
- 1 tbsp. maple syrup

Instructions:
1. Rinse the quinoa in cool water.
2. Combine quinoa and water in a saucepan. Bring to a boil, then lower to a low heat, cover, and cook for 15 minutes, or until the quinoa is tender.
3. Toss cooked quinoa with diced apples, cinnamon, chopped pecans, and maple syrup in a mixing dish.
4. Stir well and serve warm.

Nutritional Factors:
- 350 calories
- 8g protein
- 7g fiber
- 10g of good fats

Preparation Time: 20 minutes

ALZHEIMER'S DISEASE LUNCH RECIPES

1. *Salad with spinach and salmon*

Ingredients:
- 2 cups fresh spinach leaves
- 4 ounces flaked grilled salmon
- 1/2 cup halved cherry tomatoes
- 1/4 cup thinly sliced red onion
- 1/4 cup diced cucumber
- 2 tablespoons crumbled feta cheese
- 1 tablespoon olive oil
- 1 tablespoon balsamic vinegar
- Salt and pepper to taste

Instructions:
1. Toss together spinach, grilled salmon, cherry tomatoes, red onion, cucumber, and feta cheese in a large mixing bowl.
2. In a small mixing bowl, combine the olive oil, balsamic vinegar, salt, and pepper.
3. Pour the dressing over the salad and gently toss to mix.
4. Serve right away.

Nutritional Factors:
- 400 calories

- 30g protein
- 5g fiber
- 20g of good fats
- Omega-3 Fatty Acids: abundant

Time to Prepare: 15 minutes

2. Stir-Fry with Quinoa and Vegetables

Ingredients:
1 cup quinoa, 2 cups water, 1 tablespoon vegetable oil,
1 cup broccoli florets, 1 cup sliced bell peppers
- 1 cup snap peas
- 2 julienned carrots
- 2 teaspoons low-sodium soy sauce
1 teaspoon sesame oil
- 1 teaspoon minced ginger
- 1 teaspoon minced garlic
- Sesame seeds for decoration

Instructions:
1. Rinse the quinoa in cool water.
2. Combine quinoa and water in a saucepan. Bring to a boil, then lower to a low heat, cover, and cook for 15 minutes, or until the quinoa is tender.
3. Heat the vegetable oil in a large pan over medium heat.

4. Combine broccoli, bell peppers, snap peas, and carrots in a mixing bowl. Cook until the veggies are tender-crisp.
5. Stir in the cooked quinoa.
6. Combine soy sauce, sesame oil, ginger, and garlic in a small bowl. Toss the quinoa and veggies in the dressing to mix.
7. Serve garnished with sesame seeds.

Nutritional Factors:
- 450 calories
- 15g protein - 8g fiber
- 10g of good fats

Preparation Time: 25 Minutes

3. Wrap with Turkey and Avocado

Ingredients:
- 1 whole-wheat wrap
- 4 oz. sliced turkey breast
- 1/2 sliced avocado
- 1/4 cup halved cherry tomatoes
- 1 tablespoon mixed greens
- 1 tbsp. Greek yogurt
- Season with salt and pepper to taste

Instructions:
1. Place the whole-grain wrap on a clean surface and lay it flat.
2. Arrange the turkey pieces, avocado, cherry tomatoes, and mixed greens on a plate.
3. Drizzle with Greek yogurt and season with salt and pepper.
4. Tightly roll the wrap, fastening with toothpicks if required.
5. Cut into half and serve.

Nutritional Factors:
- 350 calories
- 25g protein
- 6g fiber
- 15g of good fats

Time to Prepare: 10 minutes

4. Lentil and Veggie Soup

Ingredients:
- 1 cup washed dry lentils
- 4 cups veggie broth
- 1 diced onion
- 2 sliced carrots
- 2 chopped celery stalks
- 2 minced garlic cloves
  1 can (14 oz.) chopped tomatoes

- 1 tsp cumin
- 1 tsp smoked paprika
- Season with salt and pepper to taste
- Garnish with fresh parsley

Instructions:
1. Combine lentils, vegetable broth, onion, carrots, celery, garlic, chopped tomatoes, cumin, smoked paprika, salt, and pepper in a large saucepan.
2. Bring to a boil, then lower to a low heat and continue to cook for 25-30 minutes, or until the lentils are cooked.
3. Taste for seasoning and sprinkle with fresh parsley before serving.

Nutritional Factors:
- 300 calories
- 18g protein - 12g fiber
- 2g of healthy fat

Preparation Time: 35 Minutes

5. Greek Yogurt Parfait

Ingredients:
- 1 cup plain Greek yogurt
- 1 granola cup
1/2 cup mixed berries (strawberries, blueberries)
- 1/4 cup chopped almonds - 1 tablespoon honey

Instructions:

1. Layer Greek yogurt, granola, and mixed berries in a glass or dish.
2. Drizzle with honey and sprinkle with sliced almonds.
3. Continue with the layers.
4. Serve immediately to keep the granola crunchy.

Nutritional Factors:

- 350 calories
- 20g protein
- 6g fiber
- 15g of good fats
- Probiotics: abundant

Preparation Time: 5 Minutes

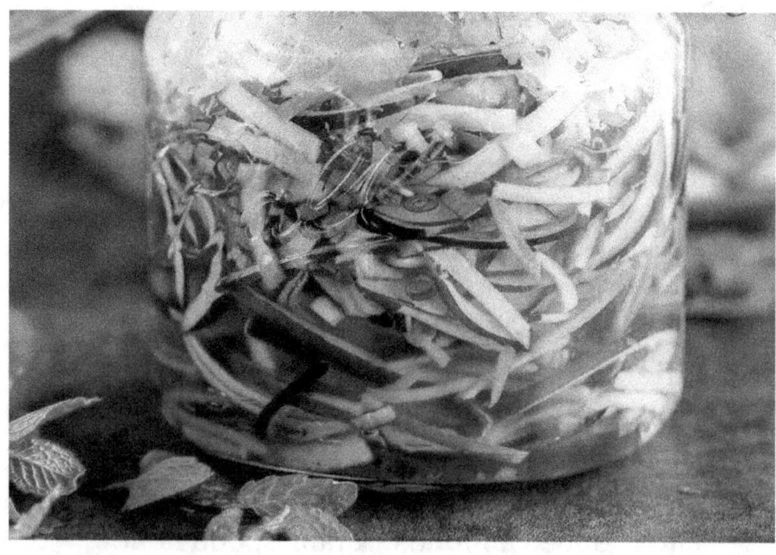

6. Bowl of Sweet Potatoes and Black Beans

Ingredients:
- 1 medium diced sweet potato
- 1 cup cooked and drained black beans
1 cup chopped kale, 1 tablespoon olive oil
1 teaspoon cumin, 1 teaspoon chili powder
- Season with salt and pepper to taste
- Top with avocado slices

Instructions:
1. Heat the oven to 400°F (200°C).
2. Combine sweet potato cubes, olive oil, cumin, chili powder, salt, and pepper in a mixing bowl.
3. Roast for 20-25 minutes, or until tender, on a baking sheet.
4. Sauté kale in a pan until wilted.
5. Toss together the roasted sweet potatoes, black beans, sautéed kale, and avocado slices in a dish.

Nutritional Factors:
- 380 calories
- 15g protein
- 10g fiber
- 10g of good fats
- Vitamin A: abundant

30 minutes of cooking time

7. Oatmeal with Almonds and Berries:

Ingredients:
- 1 cup rolled oats, old-fashioned
- 2 cups water
- 1 cup berries (blueberries, strawberries, and raspberries)
2 tbsp honey 1/4 cup chopped nuts (almonds, walnuts)
- 1/2 teaspoon ground cinnamon, 1/2 cup skim milk

Instructions:
1. Bring water to a boil in a saucepan.
2. Stir in the rolled oats and reduce to a low heat. Cook, stirring periodically, for 5-7 minutes, or until the oats are creamy.
3. Turn off the heat and stir in the mixed berries, honey, chopped almonds, cinnamon, and milk.
4. Give it a good stir and let aside for a minute to enable the berries to soften.
5. Serve warm and enjoy the nutritious delight.

Nutritional Factors:
- 400 calories
- 15g protein
- 8g fiber
- 10g of good fats
- Antioxidants: abundant

Preparation Time: 10 minutes

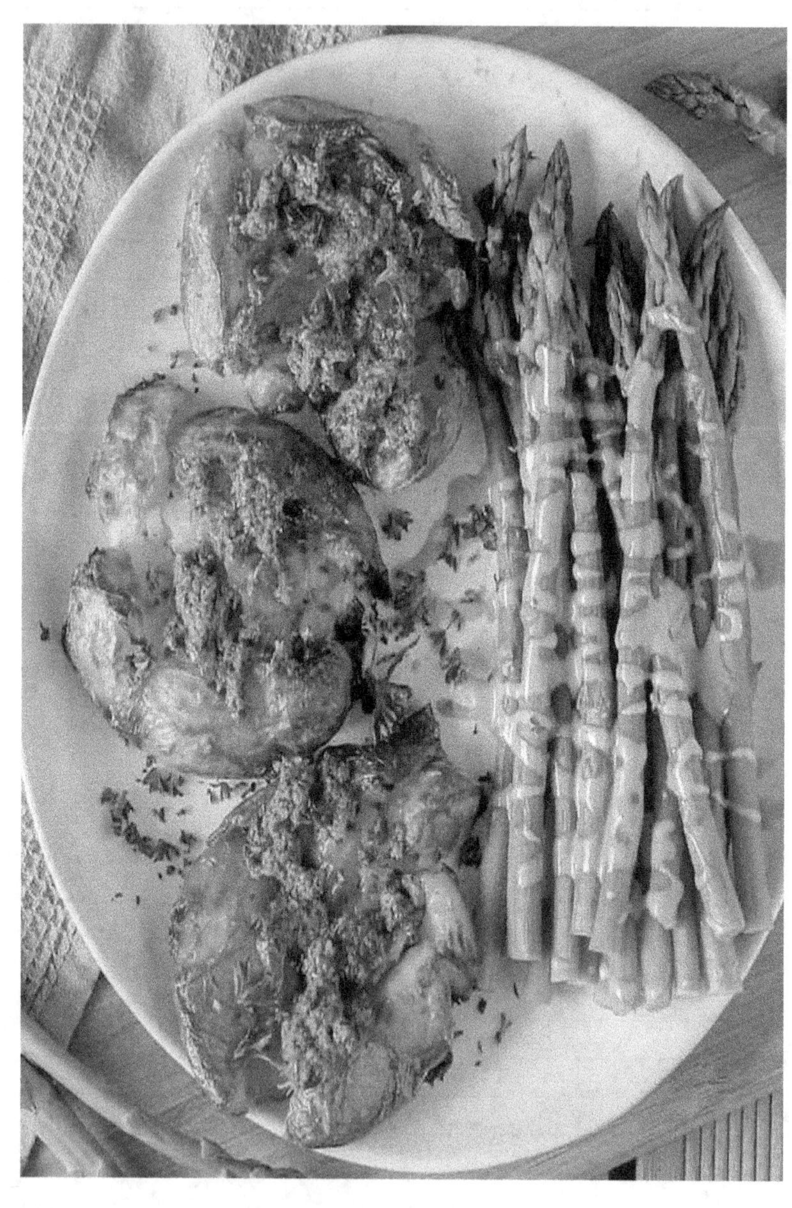

ALZHEIMER'S DISEASE DINNER RECIPES.

1. Baked Salmon and Quinoa

Ingredients:
- 4 salmon fillets (each 6 ounces)
1 cup quinoa 2 cups water or veggie broth, 1 sliced lemon
- 2 tbsp. olive oil
- 1 tsp. garlic powder
- 1 teaspoon dried thyme
- Season with salt and pepper to taste
- Garnish with fresh parsley

Instructions:
1. Preheat the oven to 375 degrees Fahrenheit (190 degrees Celsius).
2. Rinse the quinoa with cool water.
3. Combine quinoa and water or vegetable broth in a saucepan. Bring to a boil, then lower to a low heat, cover, and cook for 15 minutes, or until the quinoa is tender.
4. Line a baking sheet with parchment paper and place the salmon fillets on it.
5. Drizzle the salmon with olive oil and season with garlic powder, dried thyme, salt, and pepper.
6. Serve the salmon with lemon slices on top.

7. Bake for 15-20 minutes, or until the salmon is cooked through, in a preheated oven.
8. Serve the salmon over quinoa with fresh parsley on top.

Nutritional Factors:
- 450 calories
- 30g protein
- 5g fiber
- 20g of good fats
- Omega-3 Fatty Acids: abundant

Preparation Time: 25 Minutes

2. Mediterranean Chickpea Salad

Ingredients:
- 2 cups canned chickpeas, drained and rinsed
- 1 cup halved cherry tomatoes
- 1 diced cucumber
- 1/2 cup sliced Kalamata olives
- 1/4 cup finely chopped red onion
- 1/2 cup crumbled feta cheese
- 1/4 cup chopped fresh parsley
- 2 tbsp. olive oil
- 1 tbsp. red wine vinegar
- Season with salt and pepper to taste

Instructions:

1. Combine chickpeas, cherry tomatoes, cucumber, Kalamata olives, red onion, feta cheese, and fresh parsley in a large mixing basin.

2. In a small mixing bowl, combine the olive oil, red wine vinegar, salt, and pepper.

3. Pour the dressing over the salad and gently toss to mix.

4. Serve cold.

Nutritional Factors:

- 350 calories
- 15g protein
- 10g fiber
- 15g of good fats

Time to Prepare: 15 minutes

3 Stir-Fried Tofu with Vegetables

Ingredients:

- 1 firm tofu block, squeezed and diced
- 2 cups broccoli florets
- 1 sliced bell pepper
- 1 julienned carrot
- 2 tablespoons soy sauce, 1 teaspoon sesame oil
- 1 teaspoon minced ginger
- 1 teaspoon minced garlic
- Sesame seeds for decoration

- Chopped green onions for garnish

Instructions:
1. In a wok or large pan, heat the sesame oil over medium-high heat.
2. Stir-fry the tofu cubes until golden brown.
3. Stir in the broccoli, bell pepper, and carrot. Cook until the veggies are tender-crisp.
4. Combine soy sauce, ginger, and garlic in a small bowl. Toss the tofu and veggies in the sauce to mix.
5. Garnish with sesame seeds and green onions, if desired.
6. Plate with quinoa or brown rice.

Nutritional Factors:
- 400 calories
- 20g protein - 8g fiber
- 15g of good fats

Preparation Time: 20 minutes

4. Roasted Chicken with Sweet Potatoes

Ingredients:
- 4 boneless, skinless chicken thighs
- 2 peeled and diced sweet potatoes
- 2 tablespoons olive oil
- 1 teaspoon paprika
- 1 tsp. dried thyme

- Season with salt and pepper to taste
- Garnish with fresh rosemary

Instructions:
1. Preheat the oven to 400 degrees Fahrenheit (200 degrees Celsius).
2. Line a baking sheet with parchment paper and place the chicken thighs and sweet potato cubes on it.
3. Drizzle the chicken and sweet potatoes with olive oil.
4. Season the chicken and sweet potatoes with paprika, dried thyme, salt, and pepper.
5. Toss to evenly coat, then arrange in a single layer.
6. Bake for 40-45 minutes, or until the chicken is cooked through and the sweet potatoes are soft.
7. Before serving, garnish with fresh rosemary.

Nutritional Factors:
- 500 calories
- 30g protein - 8g fiber
- 20g of good fats

Preparation Time: 45 Minutes

5. Spinach and Mushroom Omelette

Ingredients:
- 2 eggs
- 1 cup chopped fresh spinach
- 1/2 cup sliced mushrooms, 1 teaspoon olive oil
- Season with salt and pepper to taste

Instructions:
1. In a pan over medium heat, heat the olive oil.
2. Sauté the mushrooms until tender.
3. Add the spinach and simmer until it has wilted.
4. In a mixing dish, whisk together the eggs and season with salt and pepper.
5. Pour the eggs over the veggies and gently stir until the eggs are fully cooked.
6. Serve immediately.

Nutritional Factors:
- 250 calories
- 15g protein
- 3g fiber
- 18g of healthy fat
- Vitamin K: abundant

Preparation Time: 10 minutes

6. Vegetable and Lentil Stew

Ingredients:
- 1 cup washed dry green lentils
- 4 cups veggie broth
- 1 diced onion, 2 sliced carrots
- 2 chopped celery stalks
- 2 minced garlic cloves, 1 can (14 oz.) chopped tomatoes
- 1 tsp cumin, 1 tsp smoked paprika
- Season with salt and pepper to taste
- Garnish with fresh cilantro

Instructions:
1. Combine lentils, vegetable broth, onion, carrots, celery, garlic, chopped tomatoes, cumin, smoked paprika, salt, and pepper in a large saucepan.
2. Bring to a boil, then lower to a low heat and continue to cook for 25-30 minutes, or until the lentils are cooked.
3. Taste for spice and sprinkle with fresh cilantro before serving.

Nutritional Factors:
- 350 calories
- 18g protein
- 12g fiber
- 2g of healthy fat

Preparation Time: 35 Minutes

7. Grilled Turkey Burgers with Avocado

Ingredients:
- 1/2 cup breadcrumbs, 1 pound ground turkey
- 1 egg - 1 tsp garlic powder, 1 tablespoon onion powder
- Season with salt and pepper to taste, 4 whole-grain hamburger buns
- 2 sliced avocados, For garnish, lettuce and tomato

Instructions:
1. Combine ground turkey, breadcrumbs, egg, garlic powder, onion powder, salt, and pepper in a mixing bowl. Combine thoroughly.
2. Divide the ingredients into four equal parts and form into burger patties.
3. Heat a grill or grill pan on medium-high.
4. Cook the turkey burgers for 5-7 minutes each side, or until done.
5. On the grill, toast the burger buns.
6. Top the burgers with lettuce, tomato slices, avocado slices, and your preferred condiments.
7. Serve immediately.

Nutritional Factors:
- 400 calories
- 25g protein - 6g fiber
- 15g of good fats

Preparation Time: 15 Minutes

ALZHEIMER'S DISEASE DESSERT RECIPES

1. Blueberry Oatmeal Bars

Ingredients:
-2 cups old fashioned rolled oats, 1 cup almond flour
1/2 cup melted coconut oil
- Half a cup maple syrup
- 1/2 teaspoon cinnamon
- 1 teaspoon vanilla extract
- 1 cup blueberries
- 1/4 teaspoon salt

Instructions:
1. Preheat the oven to 350 degrees Fahrenheit (175 degrees Celsius) and line a baking sheet with parchment paper.
2. Combine rolled oats, almond flour, melted coconut oil, maple syrup, vanilla extract, cinnamon, and salt in a mixing dish.
3. Spread two-thirds of the mixture in the prepared baking pan.
4. Evenly distribute the blueberries over the oat mixture.
5. Sprinkle the leftover oat mixture on top of the blueberries.

6. Bake for 25-30 minutes, or until golden brown on top.
7. Allow to cool completely before cutting into bars.

Nutritional Factors:
- 200 calories
- 4g protein
- 4g fiber
- 10g of good fats
- Antioxidants: abundant

30 minutes of cooking time

2. Chia Pudding:

Ingredients:
- 1 tablespoon chia seeds
1 cup of almond milk
- 1 tbsp honey or maple syrup
- 1/2 tsp vanilla extract
- Fresh fruit (berries, sliced banana) as a garnish

Instructions:
1. Combine chia seeds, almond milk, honey or maple syrup, and vanilla extract in a mixing dish.
2. Stir thoroughly and place in the fridge for at least 2 hours or overnight.
3. Before serving, re-stir the mixture and garnish with fresh fruit.

Nutritional Factors:
- 150 calories
- 4g protein
- 8g fiber
- 8g of healthy fat
- Omega-3 Fatty Acids: abundant

Time to Prepare: 5 minutes (plus chilling time)

3. Banana Ice Cream

Ingredients:
- 4 ripe bananas, peeled, sliced, and frozen
- 2 tbsp (optional) almond milk
- Optional toppings (nuts, dark chocolate chips, berries)

Instructions:
1. In a blender or food processor, combine frozen banana slices.
2. Puree until smooth, adding almond milk as required for a creamier texture.
3. Place in bowls or cones.
4. Garnish with your preferred healthy toppings.

Nutritional Factors:
- 150 calories
- 2g protein
- 3g fiber, 1 gram of healthy fat

Time to Prepare: 10 minutes

4 Baked Apples

Ingredients:
- 4 cored and halved apples
- 1/4 cup chopped nuts (walnuts or almonds)
- 1/2 teaspoon cinnamon
- 1 tablespoon honey

Instructions:
1. Preheat the oven to 375 degrees Fahrenheit (190 degrees Celsius).
2. Line a baking dish with apple halves.
3. Combine chopped nuts, honey, and cinnamon in a mixing dish.
4. Place a spoonful of the nut mixture in the middle of each apple half.
5. Bake for 20-25 minutes, or until the apples are soft.
6. Serve hot.

Nutritional Factors:
- 180 calories
- 2g protein
- 5g fiber
- 8g of healthy fat

Preparation Time: 25 Minutes

5. Greek Yogurt Parfait

Ingredients:
- 1 cup plain Greek yogurt
- 1 granola cup
1/2 cup mixed berries (strawberries, blueberries)
- 1/4 cup chopped almonds - 1 tablespoon honey

Instructions:
1. Layer Greek yogurt, granola, and mixed berries in a glass or dish.
2. Drizzle with honey and sprinkle with sliced almonds.
3. Continue with the layers.
4. Serve immediately to keep the granola crunchy.

Nutritional Factors:
- 350 calories
- 20g protein
- 6g fiber
- 15g of good fats
- Probiotics: abundant

Preparation Time: 5 Minutes

6. Pumpkin Chia Mousse

Ingredients:
- 1/2 cup pureed canned pumpkin
- 1/2 cup Greek yogurt
- 2 teaspoons chia seeds
-2 tbsp. honey or maple syrup
- 1/2 tsp pumpkin pie spice
- Chopped nuts for decoration

Instructions:
1. Combine pumpkin puree, Greek yogurt, chia seeds, honey or maple syrup, and pumpkin spice in a mixing bowl.
2. Stir thoroughly and place in the fridge for at least 2 hours or overnight.
3. Before serving, stir the mixture one more and sprinkle with chopped nuts.

Nutritional Factors:
- 250 calories
- 10g protein
- 8g fiber
- 10g of good fats

Time to Prepare: 5 minutes (plus chilling time)

7. Cocoa Avocado Pudding

Ingredients:
- 2 avocados, ripe
- 1/4 cup chocolate powder
- 1/4 cup maple syrup or honey
- 1/4 cup almond milk
- 1 tsp vanilla essence - pinch salt
- fresh berries for garnish

Instructions:
1. Combine avocados, cocoa powder, honey or maple syrup, almond milk, vanilla extract, and a bit of salt in a blender or food processor.
2. Blend until the mixture is smooth and creamy.
3. Transfer to serving dishes and chill for at least 30 minutes.
4. Before serving, top with fresh berries.

Nutritional Factors:
- 300 calories
- 4g protein - 8g fiber
- 20g of good fats

Time to Prepare: 10 minutes (plus chilling time)

ALZHEIMER'S DISEASE SNACKS RECIPES.

1. Blueberry-Almond Pudding:

Ingredients:
- 1 cup plain Greek yogurt
- 1/2 cup fresh blueberries
- 2 tablespoons chopped almonds
- 1 tablespoon honey

Instructions:
1. Layer Greek yogurt, blueberries, and sliced almonds in a glass or dish.
2. Drizzle with honey over top.
3. Continue with the layers.
4. Serve right away.

Nutritional Factors:
- 250 calories
- 15g protein
- 3g fiber
- 10g of good fats
- Antioxidants: abundant

Time to Prepare: 5 minutes

2. Salmon on Avocado Toast

Ingredients:
- 2 toasted slices whole-grain bread
- 1 ripe avocado, mashed
- 4 oz. smoked salmon
1 teaspoon capers
- Lemon slices for decoration

Instructions:
1. Evenly spread mashed avocado over toasted whole-grain bread.
2. Top with smoked salmon and sprinkle with capers.
3. Serve with lemon wedges as garnish.
4. Serve right away.

Nutritional Factors:
- 350 calories
- 20g protein
- 8g fiber
- 15g of good fats
- Omega-3 Fatty Acids: abundant

Time to Prepare: 10 minutes

3. Stuffed Spinach and Feta Mushrooms

Ingredients:
- 12 big mushrooms, stems removed
- 1 cup chopped fresh spinach
- 1/2 cup crumbled feta cheese
- 1 garlic clove, minced
1 teaspoon olive oil
- Season with salt and pepper to taste

Instructions:
1. Preheat the oven to 375 degrees Fahrenheit (190 degrees Celsius).
2. Heat the olive oil in a skillet over medium heat.
3. Sauté the garlic until aromatic.
4. Add the spinach and simmer until it has wilted.
5. Combine the sautéed spinach and crumbled feta in a mixing bowl.
Fill each mushroom cap with the spinach-feta mixture.
7. Arrange the filled mushrooms on a baking sheet and bake for 15-20 minutes, or until soft.
8. Serve hot.

Nutritional Factors:
- 200 calories
- 10g protein
- 5g fiber
- 15g of good fats
- Vitamin K: abundant

Preparation Time: 20 minutes

4. Nuts and Berries Trail Mix

Ingredients:
- 1/2 cup of almonds
- 1/2 cup of walnuts
- 1 tablespoon dried cranberries
- 1 tablespoon dried blueberries
- 1 tablespoon pumpkin seeds
- 1 tablespoon dark chocolate chips

Instructions:
1. Combine almonds, walnuts, dried cranberries, dried blueberries, pumpkin seeds, and dark chocolate chips in a mixing dish.
2. Toss everything together.
3. Divide the mixture into snack-sized containers for simple grab-and-go access.

Nutritional Factors:
- 400 calories
- 12g protein
- 8g fiber
- 30g of healthy fat
- Antioxidants: abundant

Time to Prepare: 5 minutes

5. Sliced cucumber with hummus

Ingredients:
- 1 sliced cucumber
- Half a cup hummus

Instructions:
1. Thinly slice the cucumber into rounds.
2. Arrange the cucumber slices on a serving platter.
3. Before eating, dip each cucumber slice into hummus.

Nutritional Factors:
- 150 calories
- 5g protein
- 4g fiber
- 10g of good fats

Time to Prepare: 5 minutes

6. Fruit Salad with Quinoa

Ingredients:
- 1 cup cooled cooked quinoa
- 1 cup fresh fruit mixture (strawberries, kiwi, pineapple, grapes)
- 2 teaspoons honey
- 1 tablespoon chopped fresh mint

Instructions:

1. In a mixing dish, combine cooked and cooled quinoa with a variety of fresh fruits.
2. Drizzle honey over the top and gently stir.
3. For extra taste, top with chopped fresh mint.
4. Serve cold.

Nutritional Factors:

- 300 calories
- 5g protein
- 6g fiber
- 3g of healthy fat
- Vitamins and minerals: abundant

Time to Prepare: 15 minutes

7. Cottage Cheese with Berries

Ingredients:

- 1 cup cottage cheese (low-fat)
- 1/2 cup berry mixture (blueberries, raspberries, strawberries)
-1 teaspoon honey

Instructions:

1. Place cottage cheese in a mixing basin.
2. Garnish with mixed berries.
3. Drizzle with honey over top.
4. Serve cold.

Nutritional Factors:

- 250 calories
- 25g protein
- 3g fiber
- 5g of healthy fat
- Antioxidants: abundant

Time to Prepare: 5 minutes

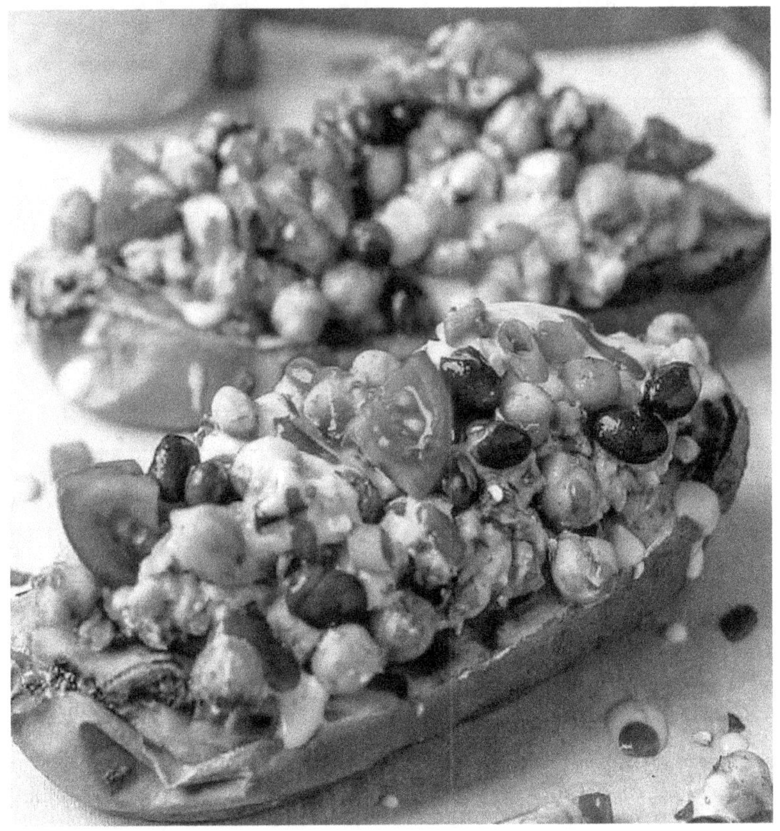

ALZHEIMER'S DISEASE SMOOTHIE RECIPES.

1. *Avocado Antioxidant Delight*

Ingredients:
- 1/2 peeled and pitted avocado
- 1/2 cup blueberries
- 1/2 cup hulled strawberries
- 1/2 cup almond milk
- 1 cup spinach
1 teaspoon chia seeds
- Optional (ice cubes)

Instructions:
1. In a blender, combine the avocado, blueberries, strawberries, spinach, almond milk, and chia seeds.
2. Blend until the mixture is smooth and creamy.
3. If desired, add ice cubes and mix again.
4. Pour into a glass and serve right away.

Nutritional Factors:
- 250 calories
- 6g protein
- 10g fiber
- 15g of good fats
- Antioxidants: abundant

Time to Prepare: 5 minutes

2. Berry Brain Boost

Ingredients:
- 1/2 banana
- 1 cup mixed berries (blueberries, raspberries, strawberries)
- 1/2 cup plain Greek yogurt
- 1 tbsp flaxseeds
- Half a cup of water or coconut water
- Optional (ice cubes)

Instructions:
1. In a blender, combine the mixed berries, banana, Greek yogurt, flaxseeds, and water.
2. Puree until smooth.
3. If desired, add ice cubes and mix again.
4. Strain into a glass and serve.

Nutritional Factors:
- 200 calories
- 8g protein
- 7g fiber
- 5g of healthy fat
- Moderate Omega-3 Fatty Acids

Time to Prepare: 5 minutes

3. Citrus Omega-Bliss

Ingredients:
- Half a cup orange juice
- Half a cup pineapple pieces
- Half a banana
- 1 tbsp. chia seeds
- 1 tbsp. hemp seeds
- 1/2 cup plain Greek yogurt
- Optional (ice cubes)

Instructions:
1. Blend together orange juice, pineapple chunks, banana, chia seeds, hemp seeds, and Greek yogurt in a blender.
2. Puree until smooth.
3. If desired, add ice cubes and mix again.
4. Strain into a glass and serve.

Nutritional Factors:
- 220 calories
- 9g protein
- 6g fiber
- 8g of healthy fat
- Omega-3 Fatty Acids: abundant

Time to Prepare: 5 minutes

4. Green Memory Elixir

Ingredients:
- 1 cup stemmed and chopped kale
- 1/2 peeled and sliced cucumber
- 1/2 cored and sliced green apple
- half a lemon, juiced
- Half a cup coconut water
-1 tbsp. spirulina powder
- Optional (ice cubes)

Instructions:
1. In a blender, combine kale, cucumber, green apple, lemon juice, coconut water, and spirulina powder.
2. Puree until smooth.
3. If desired, add ice cubes and mix again.
4. Strain into a glass and serve.

Nutritional Factors:
- 150 calories
- 5g protein
- 8g fiber
- 3g of healthy fat
- Vitamins and minerals: abundant

Time to Prepare: 5 minutes

5. Memory Magic with Coconut Almonds

Ingredients:
- 1/2 cup almond milk
- 1/2 cup coconut milk
- 1/2 banana
- 1/2 cup frozen mango pieces
- 1 tbsp. coconut oil
- 1 tbsp. almond butter
- Optional (ice cubes)

Instructions:
1. Blend together coconut milk, almond milk, frozen mango chunks, banana, coconut oil, and almond butter in a blender.
2. Puree until smooth.
3. If desired, add ice cubes and mix again.
4. Strain into a glass and serve.

Nutritional Factors:
- 300 calories
- 6g protein
- 5g fiber
- 20g of good fats
- Moderate-Medium Chain Triglycerides (MCTs):

Time to Prepare: 5 minutes

6. Spinach and Walnut Delight

Ingredients:
- 1/2 cup frozen berries (blueberries or strawberries)
- 1 cup spinach
- 1 tablespoon walnuts
- Half a banana
- 1/2 cup liquid (water or almond milk)
- 1 tbsp flaxseeds
- Optional (ice cubes)

Instructions:
1. In a blender, combine spinach, frozen berries, walnuts, banana, water or almond milk, and flaxseeds.
2. Puree until smooth.
3. If desired, add ice cubes and mix again.
4. Strain into a glass and serve.

Nutritional Factors:
- 220 calories
- 7g protein
- 8g fiber
- 12g of good fats
- Moderate Omega-3 Fatty Acids

Time to Prepare: 5 minutes

7. Brain Booster Pumpkin Pie

Ingredients:
- 1/2 banana
- 1/2 cup canned pumpkin puree
- 1/2 cup unsweetened Greek yogurt
- 1/2 tsp pumpkin pie spice
1 tbsp. chia seeds, 1/2 cup almond milk
- Optional (ice cubes)

Instructions:
1. Combine pumpkin puree, banana, and Greek yogurt in a blender.

, as well as pumpkin spice, chia seeds, and almond milk.
2. Puree until smooth.
3. If desired, add ice cubes and mix again.
4. Strain into a glass and serve.

Nutritional Factors:
- 180 calories
- 9g protein
- 7g fiber
- 5g of healthy fat

Time to Prepare: 5 minutes

ALZHEIMER'S DISEASE VEGETABLE RECIPES.

1. Quinoa-Vegetable Stir-Fry

Ingredients:
- 1 cup quinoa
- 2 cups water
- 1 tablespoon vegetable oil
- 1 sliced bell pepper
- 1 carrot, julienned
- 1 cup snap peas
- 2 garlic cloves, minced
1 teaspoon soy sauce
1 teaspoon sesame oil
- Sesame seeds for decoration

Instructions:
1. Rinse the quinoa in cool water.
2. Combine quinoa and water in a saucepan. Bring to a boil, then lower to a low heat, cover, and cook for 15 minutes, or until the quinoa is tender.
3. Heat the vegetable oil in a wok or big pan over medium-high heat.
4. Combine broccoli, bell pepper, carrot, snap peas, and garlic in a mixing bowl. Cook until the veggies are tender-crisp.
5. Stir in the cooked quinoa.

6. Combine soy sauce and sesame oil in a small dish. Toss the quinoa and veggies in the dressing to mix.
7. Serve garnished with sesame seeds.

Nutritional Factors:
- 400 calories
- 15g protein - 8g fiber
- 10g of good fats

Preparation Time: 25 Minutes

2. Spinach and Tomato Omelette

Ingredients:
- 2 eggs
- 1/2 cup chopped fresh spinach
- 1/4 cup halved cherry tomatoes
- 2 tablespoons crumbled feta cheese
- Season with salt and pepper to taste
- 1 teaspoon olive oil

Instructions:
1. Whisk eggs in a mixing basin and season with salt and pepper.
2. Melt the butter in a nonstick pan over medium heat.
3. Add the whisked eggs to the skillet.
4. Top one-half of the omelette with chopped spinach, cherry tomatoes, and feta cheese.

5. Fold the remaining half over the veggies and continue to cook until the eggs are set.
6. To serve, slide the omelette onto a dish.

Nutritional Factors:
- 300 calories
- 20g protein - 3g fiber
- 18g of healthy fat

Preparation Time: 10 minutes

3. Roasted Vegetable Medley

Ingredients:
- 2 cups chopped mixed veggies (zucchini, bell peppers, cherry tomatoes, and red onion)
- 2 teaspoons olive oil
1 tsp dried herbs (thyme, rosemary, oregano)
- Season with salt and pepper to taste

Instructions:
1. Preheat the oven to 400 degrees Fahrenheit (200 degrees Celsius).
2. Toss mixed veggies with olive oil, dry herbs, salt, and pepper in a large mixing dish.
3. Arrange the veggies in a single layer on a baking sheet.
4. Roast for 20-25 minutes, or until veggies are soft and slightly caramelized, in a preheated oven.

5. Serve with quinoa as a side dish.

Nutritional Factors:
- 200 calories
- 3g protein - 6g fiber
- 10g of good fats

Preparation Time: 25 Minutes

4. Stir-Fry Cauliflower "Rice"

Ingredients:
- 1 head shredded cauliflower
- 1 tablespoon vegetable oil
- 1 cup veggies (peas, carrots, corn)
- 2 minced garlic cloves
- 2 beaten eggs
- 2 teaspoons soy sauce
- Garnishing with green onions

Instructions:
1. Using a box grater or food processor, grate the cauliflower.
2. In a wok or big pan, heat the vegetable oil over medium-high heat.
3. Stir in the mixed veggies and garlic. Cook until the veggies are soft.
4. Push the veggies to one side of the pan and pour the beaten eggs into the other. Make the eggs scrambled.

5. Combine the scrambled eggs and veggies.

6. Stir-fry the grated cauliflower in the pan for 5-7 minutes.

7. Toss the cauliflower "rice" with the soy sauce to mix. Serve garnished with green onions.

Nutritional Factors:

- 250 calories
- 10g protein
- 8g fiber
- 12g of good fats

Preparation Time: 15 Minutes

5. Hash of Sweet Potatoes and Kale

Ingredients:

- 2 peeled and diced sweet potatoes
- 1 tablespoon olive oil
- 1 chopped onion
- 2 cups chopped kale
- 1 teaspoon smoked paprika
- Season with salt and pepper to taste

Instructions:

1. Heat the olive oil in a skillet over medium heat.

2. Add the diced sweet potatoes and cook until they soften.

3. Add the chopped onion and continue to simmer until the sweet potatoes are tender.
4. Add the greens and simmer until wilted.
5. Season the hash with smoked paprika, salt, and pepper. To mix, toss everything together.
6. Serve hot.

Nutritional Factors:
- 300 calories
- 5g protein
- 7g fiber
- Fats that are good for you: 8g

Preparation Time: 20 minutes

6. Quiche with Mushrooms and Spinach

Ingredients:
- 1 refrigerated pie crust
- 1 cup chopped mushrooms
- 2 cups fresh spinach
- 1/2 cup crumbled feta cheese
- 4 eggs
- 1 cup of milk
- To taste, salt and pepper
- 1/2 teaspoon dried thyme

Instructions:

1. Preheat the oven to 375 degrees Fahrenheit (190 degrees Celsius).

2. Roll out the pie dough and line a pie plate with it.

3. Sauté mushrooms in a pan until browned.

4. Cook until the spinach has wilted in the skillet.

5. Cover the pie shell with the mushroom and spinach mixture. Sprinkle with feta cheese.

6. Whisk together the eggs, milk, salt, pepper, and dried thyme in a mixing dish.

7. Pour the egg mixture into the pie crust over the veggies and cheese.

8. Bake for 30-35 minutes, or until the quiche is set, in a preheated oven.

Allow it cool completely before slicing and serving.

Nutritional Factors:

- 350 calories
- 15g protein
- 3g fiber
- 20g of good fats

Preparation Time: 35 Minutes

7. Stuffed Broccoli and Cheese Peppers

Ingredients:
- 4 bell peppers, halved and seeds removed
- 2 cups cooked broccoli florets
- 1 cup cooked quinoa
- 1 cup shredded cheddar cheese
- 1/2 cup plain Greek yogurt
- Season with salt and pepper to taste

Instructions:
1. Preheat the oven to 375 degrees Fahrenheit (190 degrees Celsius).
2. Steam the broccoli until it is tender-crisp.
3. Combine steamed broccoli, cooked quinoa, shredded cheddar cheese, Greek yogurt, salt, and pepper in a mixing dish.
4. Stuff each half of a bell pepper with the broccoli and cheese mixture.
5. Arrange the peppers in a baking tray.
6. Bake for 20-25 minutes, or until the peppers are cooked, in a preheated oven.
7. Serve immediately.

Nutritional Factors:
- 300 calories
- 15g protein - 8g fiber
- 10g of good fats

Preparation Time: 25 Minutes

8. Salad with Brussels Sprouts and Walnuts

Ingredients:
- 1 pound trimmed and halved Brussels sprouts
- 2 tablespoons olive oil
- 1 cup chopped walnuts
- 1/4 cup dried cranberries
- 1/4 cup crumbled feta cheese
- 2 teaspoons balsamic vinegar
- Season with salt and pepper to taste

Instructions:
1. Preheat the oven to 400 degrees Fahrenheit (200 degrees Celsius).
2. Season Brussels sprouts with salt & pepper.
3. Place the Brussels sprouts on a baking sheet and bake for 20-25 minutes, or until golden brown.
4. Toss together roasted Brussels sprouts, chopped walnuts, dried cranberries, and crumbled feta cheese in a mixing dish.
5. Drizzle the salad with balsamic vinegar and toss to mix.
6. Serve warm or at room temperature.

Nutritional Factors:

- 350 calories
- 10g protein
- 8g fiber
- 25g of good fats

Preparation Time: 25 Minutes

9. Vegetable and Lentil Soup

Ingredients:
- 1 cup washed dry green lentils
- 4 cups veggie broth - 1 diced onion
- 2 sliced carrots
- 2 chopped celery stalks
- 2 minced garlic cloves
1 can (14 oz.) chopped tomatoes
- 1 tsp cumin - 1 tsp smoked paprika
- Season with salt and pepper to taste - Garnish with fresh cilantro

Instructions:
1. Combine lentils, vegetable broth, onion, carrots, celery, garlic, chopped tomatoes, cumin, smoked paprika, salt, and pepper in a large saucepan.
2. Bring to a boil, then lower to a low heat and continue to cook for 25-30 minutes, or until the lentils are cooked.
3. Taste for spice and sprinkle with fresh cilantro before serving.

Nutritional Factors:
- 350 calories
- 18g protein - 12g fiber
- 2g of healthy fat

Preparation Time: 35 Minutes

SOME STANDARD KITCHEN MEASUREMENTS AND THEIR EQUIVALENCE.

Here are some standard kitchen measurements and their corresponding values, essential for brain/mind diet recipes

1. Teaspoon (tsp)

- Equal to 5 milliliters (ml)
- Typically employed for modest quantities of spices, extracts, or fluid elements like honey.

2. Tablespoon (tbsp)

- Equal to 15 milliliters (ml) or 3 teaspoons
- Utilized for more substantial amounts of ingredients such as condiments, oils, or sauces.

3. Cup

- Equal to 240 milliliters (ml)
- A conventional measure for both dry and liquid components like flour, sugar, or milk.

4. Fluid Ounce (Fl oz)

- Equal to 30 milliliters (ml)
- Utilized for gauging liquids such as water, juice, or milk.

5. Pint

- Equal to 16 fluid ounces or roughly 473 milliliters
- Commonly used for quantifying liquids in larger volumes.

6. Quart

- Equal to 32 fluid ounces or approximately 946 milliliters
- Frequently employed for more substantial liquid volumes in cooking or baking.

7. Gallon

- Equal to 128 fluid ounces or about 3,785 milliliters
- A larger unit applied for measuring bulk liquid volumes.

8. Ounce (oz)

- Equal to approximately 28.35 grams
- Utilized for measuring both dry and liquid ingredients, particularly in smaller amounts.

9. Pound (lb.)

- Equal to 16 ounces or roughly 453.592 grams
- Typically used for measuring larger quantities of ingredients like flour, sugar, or meat.

10. Gram (g)

- A metric unit of weight, frequently used for precision in measurements.

- Approximately 28.35 grams make up one ounce.

11. Milligram (mg)
- A smaller unit of weight, especially beneficial for measuring supplements or specific additives.
- One gram is equivalent to 1,000 milligrams.

These standardized kitchen measurements play a pivotal role in accurately executing brain/mind diet recipes, ensuring precise ingredient quantities for optimal nutritional outcomes.

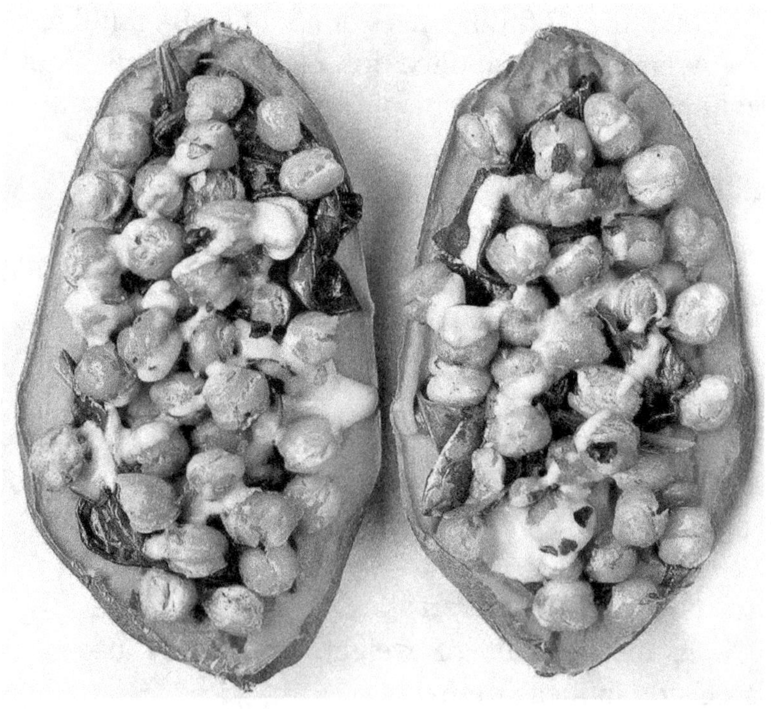

CONCLUSION

In crafting this Alzheimer's disease cookbook, our aim has been to provide not just a collection of recipes but a comprehensive guide for individuals and their caregivers navigating the challenges of Alzheimer's. Recognizing the profound impact that nutrition can have on cognitive health, we've curated a 7-day serial meal plan filled with nutrient-dense, brain-supporting foods.

These recipes emphasize a balance of omega-3 fatty acids, antioxidants, and essential nutrients found in fruits, vegetables, lean proteins, and whole grains. We've considered the challenges that may arise—both in terms of cognitive function and physical abilities— and strived to create meals that are not only nutritious but also accessible and enjoyable.

Meal planning for Alzheimer's extends beyond sustenance; it's about creating a routine that fosters predictability, reducing anxiety for individuals with Alzheimer's. The inclusion of familiar and finger-friendly foods enhances the dining experience, promoting a positive relationship with food.

As you embark on this dietary journey, we encourage you to view it not as a restrictive regimen but as a celebration of vibrant, wholesome ingredients. Adapt these recipes to suit individual tastes, dietary restrictions, and cultural preferences. Flexibility is key, and consulting with healthcare professionals ensures that the meal plan aligns seamlessly with specific health needs.

To our readers, we offer a special motivation. The commitment to this Alzheimer's diet is a powerful act of love and care, fostering not only physical health but also emotional well-being. Each thoughtfully prepared meal is a testament to the dedication to a higher quality of life, both for those with Alzheimer's and their devoted caregivers.

In closing, we express our deepest gratitude for entrusting us with this culinary journey. As you explore these recipes, savor the moments shared around the table, and witness the positive impact on cognitive health, remember that every meal is a step toward a healthier, more vibrant life.

Thank you for embracing this journey with us. Don't forget to share your thoughts and experiences with these recipes—your feedback is invaluable in continually refining and improving this resource for the benefit of others. Bon appétit, and may each bite be a nourishing step toward a brighter tomorrow.

THANK YOU!!!

IF YOU FIND THIS BOOK TO BE INFORMATIVE, INSPIRING, OR SIMPLY ENJOYABLE, I WOULD BE IMMENSELY GRATEFUL IF YOU COULD SHARE YOUR THOUGHTS WITH OTHERS. YOUR HONEST REVIEW CAN MAKE A DIFFERENCE IN HELPING MORE INDIVIDUALS DISCOVER THE BENEFITS OF A NOURISHING AND MINDFUL APPROACH TO EATING. PLEASE CONSIDER LEAVING A REVIEW ON AMAZON AND SHARE YOUR EXPERIENCE.

THANK YOU ONCE AGAIN FOR CHOOSING THIS BOOK AS A COMPANION ON YOUR PATH TO A HEALTHIER, HAPPIER YOU.

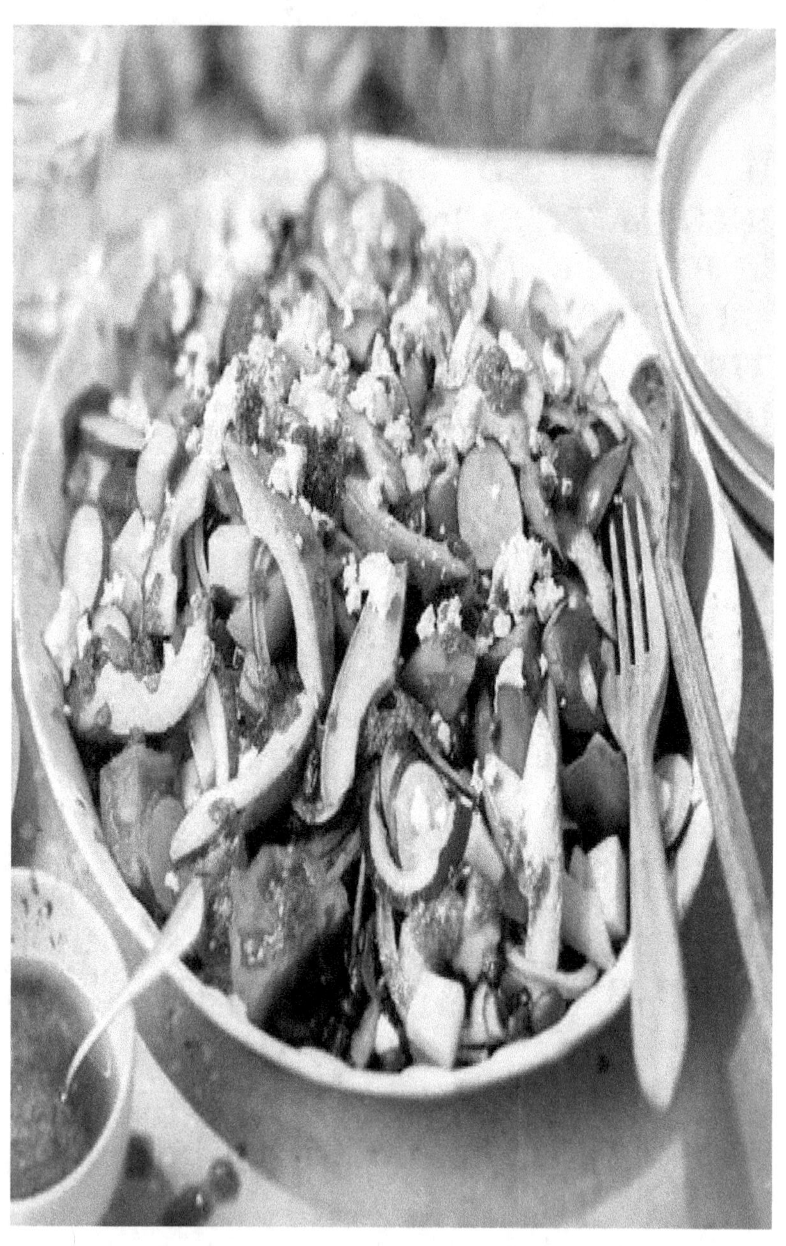

14 WEEKS ALZHEIMER'S DIET MEAL PLANNER

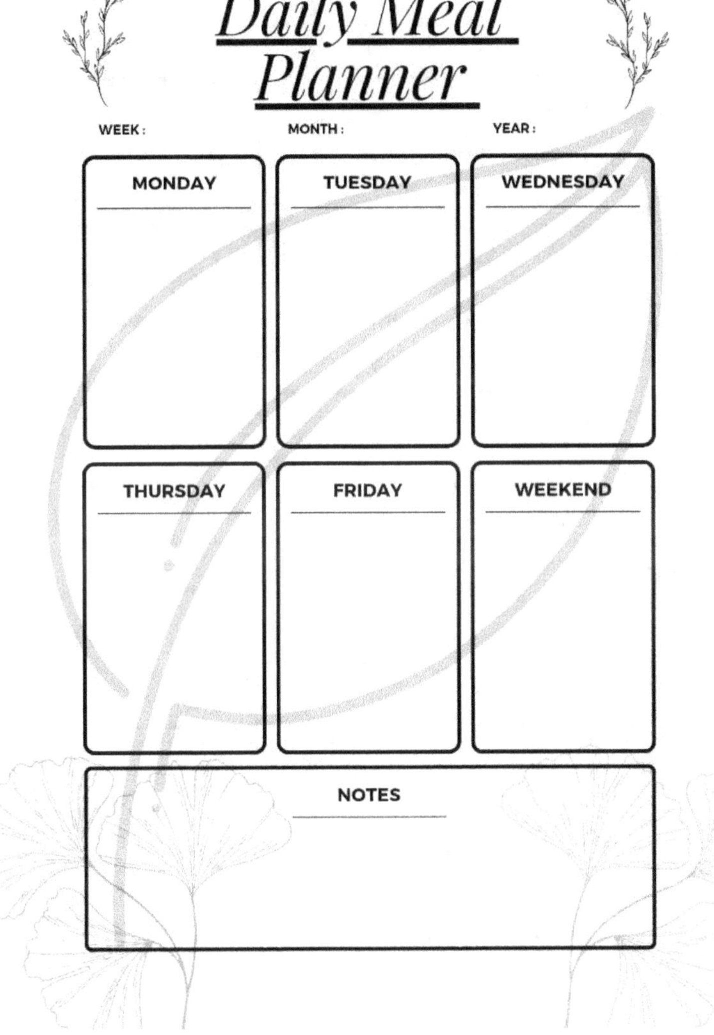

Daily Meal Planner

WEEK :   MONTH :   YEAR :

MONDAY	TUESDAY	WEDNESDAY

THURSDAY	FRIDAY	WEEKEND

NOTES

Daily Meal Planner

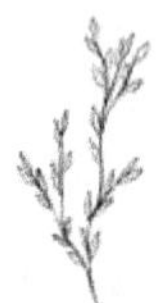 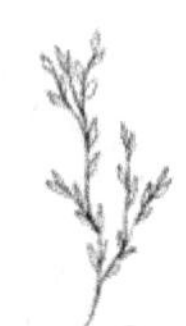

WEEK :   MONTH :   YEAR :

MONDAY	TUESDAY	WEDNESDAY

THURSDAY	FRIDAY	WEEKEND

NOTES

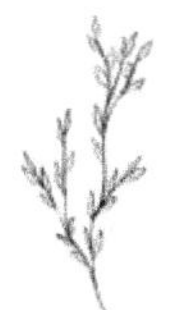
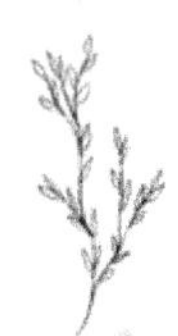

Daily Meal Planner

WEEK: **MONTH:** **YEAR:**

MONDAY	TUESDAY	WEDNESDAY

THURSDAY	FRIDAY	WEEKEND

NOTES

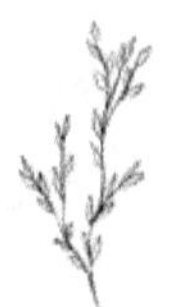 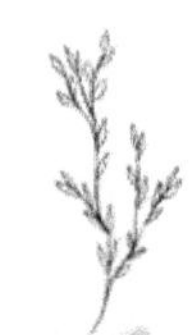

Daily Meal Planner

WEEK :   MONTH :   YEAR :

MONDAY	TUESDAY	WEDNESDAY

THURSDAY	FRIDAY	WEEKEND

NOTES

Daily Meal Planner

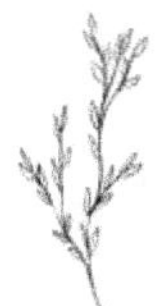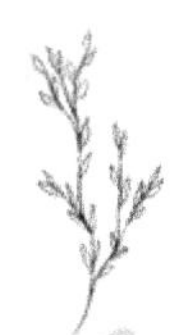

WEEK: **MONTH:**   **YEAR:**

MONDAY	TUESDAY	WEDNESDAY

THURSDAY	FRIDAY	WEEKEND

NOTES

Daily Meal Planner

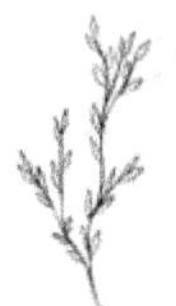 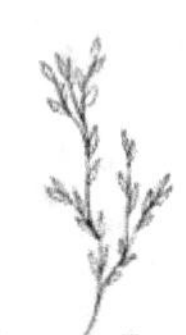

WEEK: **MONTH:** **YEAR:**

MONDAY	TUESDAY	WEDNESDAY

THURSDAY	FRIDAY	WEEKEND

NOTES

Daily Meal Planner

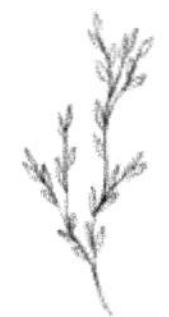
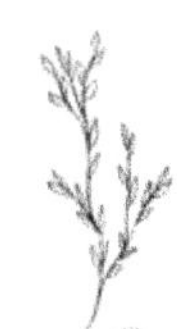

MONDAY	TUESDAY	WEDNESDAY

THURSDAY	FRIDAY	WEEKEND

NOTES

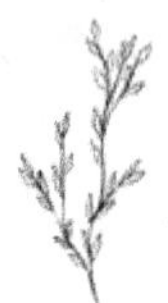
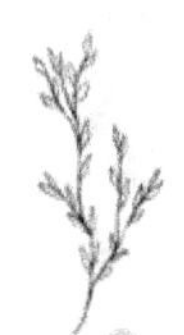

Daily Meal Planner

WEEK: MONTH: YEAR:

MONDAY	TUESDAY	WEDNESDAY

THURSDAY	FRIDAY	WEEKEND

NOTES

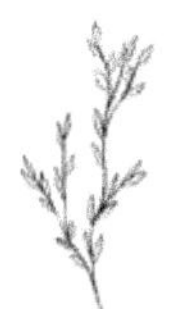
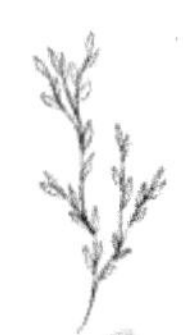

Daily Meal
Planner

WEEK : **MONTH :** **YEAR :**

MONDAY	TUESDAY	WEDNESDAY

THURSDAY	FRIDAY	WEEKEND

NOTES

Daily Meal Planner

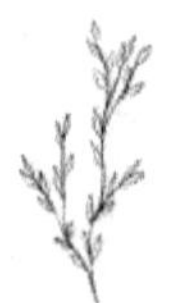
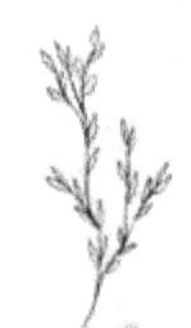

WEEK :   **MONTH :**   **YEAR :**

MONDAY	TUESDAY	WEDNESDAY

THURSDAY	FRIDAY	WEEKEND

NOTES

Daily Meal Planner

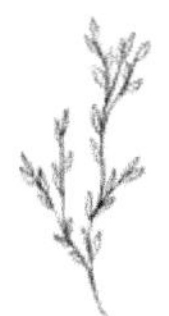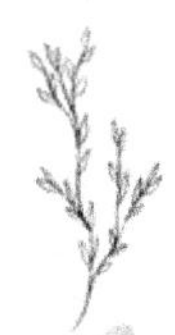

WEEK: MONTH: YEAR:

MONDAY	TUESDAY	WEDNESDAY

THURSDAY	FRIDAY	WEEKEND

NOTES

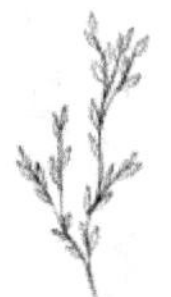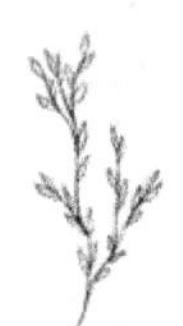

Daily Meal
Planner

WEEK :   **MONTH :**   **YEAR :**

MONDAY	TUESDAY	WEDNESDAY

THURSDAY	FRIDAY	WEEKEND

NOTES

Daily Meal Planner

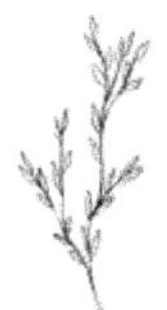

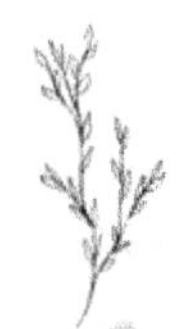

WEEK: **MONTH:**   **YEAR:**

MONDAY	TUESDAY	WEDNESDAY

THURSDAY	FRIDAY	WEEKEND

NOTES

Daily Meal Planner

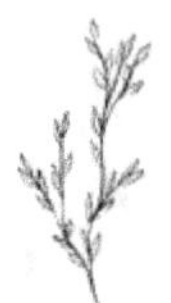
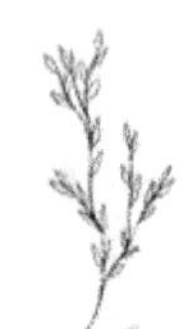

WEEK: MONTH: YEAR:

MONDAY

TUESDAY

WEDNESDAY

THURSDAY

FRIDAY

WEEKEND

NOTES